Epilepsy: A Team Approach to Effective Management

Linda Baddeley RGN MA

Clinical Nurse Specialist in Epilepsy, North Staffordshire Hospital, UK

Simon Ellis MD

Visiting Professor of Neuroscience, Staffordshire University, UK

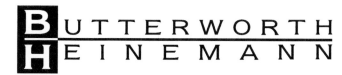

BUTTERWORTH
HEINEMANN

OXFORD AUCKLAND BOSTON JOHANNESBURG MELBOURNE NEW DELHI

Butterworth-Heinemann
Linacre House, Jordan Hill, Oxford OX2 8DP
225 Wildwood Avenue, Woburn, MA 01801-2041
A division of Reed Educational and Professional Publishing Ltd

A member of the Reed Elsevier plc group

First published 2002

British Library Cataloguing in Publication Data
Baddeley, Linda
    Epilepsy: a team approach to effective management
    1. Epilepsy – Nursing
    I. Title   II. Ellis, Simon J.
    616.8′53

ISBN 0 7506 4954 2

For information on all Butterworth-Heinemann publications
visit our website at www.bh.com

Typeset by Avocet Typeset, Brill, Aylesbury, Bucks
Printed and bound in Great Britain

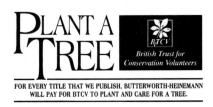

FOR EVERY TITLE THAT WE PUBLISH, BUTTERWORTH-HEINEMANN
WILL PAY FOR BTCV TO PLANT AND CARE FOR A TREE.

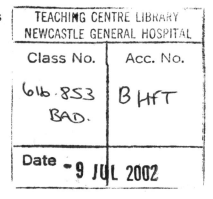

Contents

Epilepsy: A Team Approach to Effective Management

Commissioning editor: Mary Seager
Development editor: Caroline Savage
Production controller: Chris Jarvis
Desk editor: Jackie Holding
Cover designer: Gregory Harris

Preface

This book as been written to try to help provide an insight into the complexities of the diagnosis, treatment and management of epilepsy from a medical perspective. The target audience is predominantly nurses, though we hope that health care professionals from many other backgrounds may find the book will help to improve their knowledge and understanding of the medical and social implications of the condition on an individual life. It is hoped that this will not only act as a text book about epilepsy but will also provide practical working models which can be adapted for use not only in primary and secondary care but also the private sector. The intentions of the authors are to show that you do not need to be working within this specialized field to help in improving standards of care for people with epilepsy.

Epilepsy is a common condition affecting approximately 1 in 200 of the population; it is twice as common as insulin-dependant diabetes. Many people with epilepsy will have co-morbidity, or may develop unassociated medical problems; this means that nurses working in many differing areas of care may be involved in their treatment but not always because of the epilepsy. We hope to provide an insight into how any nurse involved in a patient's care, for whatever reason, can make a difference.

The book progresses through the history and social background of the condition before discussing the processes involved in making the diagnosis and the pitfalls of misdiagnosis. Some of the more common causes of epilepsy are covered including the incidence of epilepsy following neurosurgical procedures. The anatomy and biochemistry of epilepsy and the process of classifying seizures is discussed, before moving on to treatment options. In this section the main emphasis is on the use of medication and information on the different anti-epileptic drugs available, though other forms of treatment, including surgery and complimentary therapies, are covered. The potential for litigation if a misdiagnosis is made, or incorrect information supplied is also included.

The social implications of epilepsy and the impact on different age groups and sexes is an important part of this book with specific chapters covering lifestyle implications, children and adolescents, the elderly and people with learning disabilities and psychiatric problems. One chapter concentrates on the potential impact on sexuality and family planning, including problems relating to epilepsy and pregnancy.

It is because of this potential for the condition to impact at any stage in a person's life that the authors have tried to give examples of how different sections of the nursing profession can be involved in the patient's care. The aim is to reduce the morbidity of the condition and also the impact that it may have on the person's ability to deal with other problems. The authors hope that by encouraging more involvement many aspects of care can become proactive instead of reactive.

The appendices provide examples of basic patient information sheets, documentation that can be used for improving record-keeping, and also suggestions for undertaking audit to establish any need for change within a particular area of care. A protocol for the use of rectal diazepam designed by Linda Baddeley and a pharmacist, now adopted and widely used locally, is also included along with some useful addresses.

The authors hope that by showing how various health care professionals can make a difference this will help people with epilepsy get the improved service they have so long deserved.

Linda Baddeley
Colin Ellis

Acknowledgements

We would like to thank the citizens of North Staffordshire who have epilepsy and from whom it has been our privilege to know and learn. Many of our patients are stoical in the extreme and have a down-to-earth approach to getting on with life despite great difficulties.

We would also like to thank our colleagues who have supported the epilepsy service in North Staffordshire, even when it looked as though chronic under-funding was going to sink us.

As the nursing half of this double act, I (LB) would like to thank the medical and nursing staff who have been prepared to share their knowledge and expertise to help me develop the role of clinical nurse specialist locally. It is the experiences I have gained within this post that I now hope will be of some help to other professionals and encourage them to be active in improving epilepsy care within their area of work.

Many thanks to Sonia De Gannes, who has kept us more or less on time and has reviewed the manuscript. We would also like to thank all those at Butterworth-Heinemann, particularly Mary Seager, who must have found us a pain, but did not let on.

Unfortunately, due to her untimely and tragic death we cannot thank Ann Watson for her pharmaceutical advice. She will be greatly missed.

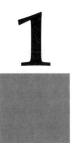

1

An introduction to epilepsy: the condition and the care

THE AIM OF THIS BOOK

The aim of this book is to increase the knowledge and understanding, for all levels of nurses and other health care professionals, of epilepsy, its diagnosis, treatment and management.

All health care professionals are likely to come into contact with patients who have epilepsy or some other seizure disorder. Nurses, in particular, in any branch of the profession need to be prepared to meet the needs of patients who have had seizures. Knowledge of the condition may not seem immediately vital to the care that you are giving, but improving your knowledge may help to improve your overall standard of care to the individual.

A better understanding of patients' epilepsy may help in your understanding of their methods of coping with other conditions, associated or coincidental.

THE SOCIAL HISTORY OF EPILEPSY

Epilepsy is the oldest known medical condition with a history of misunderstanding, misinterpretation and confusion. It was first documented at the time of the Babylonians, 2000 BC. They described attacks that today could be classified as epileptiform. However, they attributed each seizure type to being possessed by a different evil spirit or god. The Babylonians had laws that stated that these people could not marry and could not appear in court. In 400 BC, Hypocrites taught of a condition that he named from the Greek word *epilepsia*, meaning to seize or attack. He described this as having a physical rather than a spiritual cause, and not as being possessed by the devil. From these times until the twentieth century, the beliefs alternated between seeing this as a medical or a spiritual problem. Sufferers were persecuted or revered throughout time because of the misunderstanding of this condition. Reactions often depended on the culture, creed and prejudices of the societies in which they lived. Some were burned at the stake, publicly beaten or ostracized, while in other communities they were treated as gods or prophets.

Famous people thought to have had epilepsy:

- Alexander the Great
- Joan of Arc
- Julius Caesar
- George Fredrick Handel
- Van Gough
- Socrates

However, most people with epilepsy are ordinary people trying to live their lives rather than conquer the world!

In modern times we feel that our understanding and tolerance is much improved, but how far have we come? In 1857 the first drug for the treatment of epilepsy was used, yet it was only in 1970 that the United Kingdom repealed a law preventing people with epilepsy from marrying; the same law was not repealed in some states in the USA until 1980. Until 1956, in 18 states in the USA, provisions existed for the eugenic sterilization of people with epilepsy. In 1996 in the Netherlands, a man was publicly whipped and put into isolation because he had epilepsy. In India and China, developing epilepsy is still grounds for having a marriage annulled. People still talk of the reputation of the 'epilepsy colonies', which they think of along with the old workhouses and 'mental hospitals'. Even in this new millennium it is unusual for famous people to admit that they have epilepsy.

It is from this background that people with epilepsy are trying to establish some better understanding of their condition by others. This is often made more difficult because of the continued misunderstanding of the condition, even in the twenty-first century.

THE MEDICAL HISTORY OF EPILEPSY

This is no less chequered than the social history. The diagnosis of this condition has always been problematic. Even in this age of advanced technology, the most important diagnostic tool still remains the ability to listen to and interpret information supplied by the patient and any witnesses of the episodes being experienced. Diagnosis therefore remains reliant on the clinical expertise and understanding of the health care professionals.

In 1857, potassium bromide was first used to treat seizures. This was not because of any understanding of its now recognized anticonvulsant properties, but because of it's induced temporary impotence. It was believed at that time that an increased sexual drive and excessive masturbation caused seizures.

In France, demonstrations of ladies 'swooning' were used in order to show medical students the nature of seizures. These episodes would almost certainly have been induced by hyperventilation or be vaso-vagal in origin, as the ladies seemed to be able to perform to order. Many of the terms used to describe these events are still used today: *déjà vu, petit mal* and *grand mal*.

In the early nineteenth century, epilepsy was first identified as a symptom of some underlying cause. Hughlings Jackson first described an episode, experienced by his wife, of repetitive uncontrolled movements of one limb. This type of seizure became known as Jacksonian epilepsy. This remained a recognized type of epilepsy until the reclassification of seizures by the International League Against Epilepsy in 1982, and these seizures are now known as focal motor seizures. Progress in the understanding and treatment of epilepsy changed very little until the twentieth century. The introduction of electroencephalography, and radiological advances in computerized tomography and, more recently, magnetic resonance scanning, has helped to increase the understanding of cerebral function. In the last two decades research has led to better understanding of the chemical chain of events involved in the action potentials of the neurones, so helping with advancement of treatment techniques. The most recently available investigations of positron emission tomography (PET) and single photon emission computed tomography (SPECT) scans using heat-registering technology are further aiding in diagnosis of localized lesions that give rise to seizures.

THE HISTORY OF EPILEPSY THERAPY

Most of the drugs used for treating epilepsy were discovered accidentally. We have already explained about the use (or misuse) of bromides in the early treatment, but how much better understood were later drugs?

In 1912, phenobarbitone was first used as an anticonvulsant. Although it was thought to correct the electrical changes that happened during a seizure, the actual mode of action was not understood. The sedation and cognitive impairment associated with this drug are now well recognized. Long-term use is also associated with an increased incidence of osteoporosis. These days it is rarely used as a drug of choice for the newly diagnosed, although it is probably still one of the most effective treatments. Phenobarbitone is still the most commonly used drug for treating epilepsy in the Third World because of its low cost.

Phenytoin was first introduced in 1938, and was followed in 1945 by ethosuximide and then in 1952 by primidone, which was thought to be revolutionary. What was not recognized was that when this drug was metabolized it changed to phenobarbitone, therefore increasing its serum levels when the two were combined. The development of other anticonvulsant medication was slow, with no other drugs being licensed until carbamazepine in 1965, and sodium valproate in 1973.

There was then little change in the development of new drug treatment until the late 1980s and 1990s, when vigabatrin, lamotrigine, gabapentin, felbamate and topiramate were licensed. The development of new anticonvulsant continued with tiagabine and, more recently, phosphenytoin, and oxcarbazepine and levetiracetam. The problems of understanding the mechanism of seizures and the mode of action of drugs continue. Although some drugs were named because of the receptor site on which they were thought to act, e.g. gabapentin on the GABA receptors, subsequently the mode of action was found to be different from that first supposed.

Many of the older drugs are no longer in favour because of unacceptable idiosyncratic and long-term side effects, and also because of the problems with teratogenicity. They have been replaced by the 'cleaner', newer drugs, but are they indeed 'cleaner'? Already problems are being identified with some of these, resulting in their withdrawal from use (e.g. felbamate because of the risk of aplastic anaemia) or their restricted use (e.g. vigabatrin, which has been associated with visual field defects resulting in tunnel vission). Others such as lamotrigine and gabapentin also have problems that are becoming more obvious the longer they are in use. These issues will be covered in more detail in Chapter 7.

Drugs are not the only treatment for epilepsy. For some time now various surgical procedures have been used for the treatment of epilepsy, and recently there has been the introduction of vagal nerve stimulation.

With the improved understanding of this condition, the use of complementary therapies such as relaxation, aromatherapy, and diversion techniques now also play an important role in treatment. Alternative therapies will be covered in Chapter 7.

THE INCIDENCE AND PREVALENCE OF EPILEPSY

Epilepsy is the most common serious neurological condition. The reported incidence (the number of people who are newly diagnosed in 1 year) is approximately 50–80 per 100 000, while cases of single seizure are as high as 20 per 100 000. It is estimated that there are approximately 350 000 people with epilepsy in the United Kingdom.

The prevalence (the total number of people in the population with the condition) of epilepsy is reported to be approximately 5–10 per 1000. General practitioners in the UK are each estimated to have 10–15 patients with active epilepsy in their care, and potentially one or two newly diagnosed patients per year.

The highest incidence of epilepsy has previously been in children; however, recent information indicates that this age group now represents approximately 25 per cent of new cases. The increase in the elderly population and the increasing prevalence of improved cerebrovascular disease is reflected in recent research, which indicates that around 25 per cent of new cases now occur in the elderly population. In the population with a learning disability, approximately 1600 per 10 000 (16 per cent) will have epilepsy.

MORTALITY ASSOCIATED WITH EPILEPSY

It is only in recent years that the increased risk of early death has been associated with epilepsy. The risk of dying during a seizure due to status epilepticus – continuous uncontrollable seizures – has long been accepted, although other causes of deaths related to epilepsy have only more recently been recognized. These include accidental death due to drowning or burns, head injury, suicide and sudden unexplained death. The mortality rate is thought to be two to three times higher in people with epilepsy than in the general population.

A hospital study undertaken in the UK in 1995 reported the incidence of mortality in people with chronic epilepsy to be 4.5 times higher than the general population. Approximately 50 per cent of these were categorized as sudden unexpected death. The mortality rate in children with severe epilepsy and learning disability was reported in a UK audit undertaken in 1995 to be 15.9 times higher than anticipated.

The increased mortality in newly diagnosed patients is more frequently associated with an underlying cause (tumour, infection) than with the epilepsy. In people with chronic epilepsy, the death will be more likely to be associated with a seizure. In a recent obstetric audit, epilepsy was reported to be the second greatest cause of maternal death. The epilepsy task force report that in 1992, the number of deaths related to epilepsy in Britain was reported to be 900; however, this is thought to be an underestimation of the true figure.

In 1999, Epilepsy Bereaved lobbied for an audit looking at epilepsy-related deaths. This has now been approved by the Department of Health (The National Sentinel Audit). Reporting to this audit has to be done by the family via Epilepsy Bereaved, who then collect the relative information. When results are available, it is hoped that this will provide more accurate data regarding the causes of deaths and may help towards improving preventative measures and so reduce mortality. These data will again just represent a sample, as only approximately 26 per cent of coroners were thought to be taking part in the audit.

THE COST OF EPILEPSY TO THE UNITED KINGDOM

The cost of the epilepsy service within the United Kingdom in 1989 was reported to be approximately £500 million per annum. In 1998, it was estimated to be almost £2 billion per annum. These costs include not only those of direct care, but also the loss of earnings and cost of financial benefits. With the increasing cost of investigations, new anticonvulsant therapy and surgical intervention, along with the introduction of specialist nurse services and the recognized need for physiological support, the cost will continue to rise. These issues must, however, be considered against the improved standard of treatment and the increasing number of people attaining a seizure-free state, which helps them to remain independent and reduces social costs (i.e. less unemployment).

THE AETIOLOGY OF EPILEPSY

By definition, epilepsy is a state of recurrent episodes of altered or loss of consciousness. These episodes are unpredictable in their pattern of occurrence, although they are usually stereo-typed in nature in an individual (the same sort of attack occurs again and again in that person).

The epilepsy may be symptomatic, due to an underlying structural lesion. This lesion may be life threatening, or may be due to an abnormality caused by problems during foetal development. It may be cryptogenic, having no identifiable underlying cause, or it may be genetic in origin (idiopathic). Treatment is needed to any underlying cause if appropriate, or to stop the seizures in cryptogenic or idiopathic epilepsy.

The most common causes of epilepsy include:

- Trauma due to birth injury or open or closed head injury
- Cerebral infection
- Cerebrovascular events
- Cerebral tumours
- Genetic disorders
- Drug and alcohol abuse
- Other medical conditions such as multiple sclerosis and dementia.

In approximately 65 per cent of people with epilepsy, no underlying cause will be found. In most cases we are aiming to treat the symptom – the seizure – but are not able to treat the cause.

The different types of seizures that present in epilepsy will be discussed in Chapter 6.

Despite the recent improvements in investigative techniques and increasing knowledge and understanding of epilepsy, there is still much progress to be made in order to bring services in line with those of conditions such as diabetes and asthma. Nurses are in a prime position to move this standard of care forward. Epilepsy is a common condition; all health care professionals will at some time come into contact with a person with epilepsy. We do not all need to become experts, but by sharing information and care we can improve the service we provide. The role of the nurse has always been that of an educator as well as a carer. If we all improve our knowledge of epilepsy, then standards of care will also improve, and informed people can make choices that are sensible for them. Educating people empowers them, but first we must have a secure knowledge base from which we can impart information.

2 The development of epilepsy services

INTRODUCTION

In this chapter we will discuss the development of epilepsy services and try to identify some of the reasons for the slow progress until the last decade. We will also consider recent developments that may have contributed to current progress.

People with epilepsy are stigmatized. In the nineteenth century, the misconception of people with epilepsy having a learning disability or a mental health problem led to many of them being placed in 'lunatic asylums'. This was partly due to ignorance and partly because of fear within the community. The lack of medication meant that families could not cope with the uncontrolled seizures, and the practice of placing people with epilepsy in asylums was similar to that of institutionalizing unmarried mothers to save the family from disgrace. In the early twentieth century, 'epilepsy colonies' were established. The idea was to provide a sheltered environment in which people with severe epilepsy could live and work, although they still encouraged segregation from the family and were usually based on single-sex units. Many of the people within these colonies had no problems other than their uncontrolled epilepsy. Although we now criticize such institutions, at the time this may have been a better option than leaving people with epilepsy living with families who could not cope, and in a society that did not understand and was often not willing to accept anyone that it did not consider 'normal'. Many people with epilepsy did lead ordinary lives; they worked, married, had families and were part of the community. However, these people were able to hide their seizures from others, and it was not uncommon for other members of the family, even husband and wives, to be unaware of the condition. In some cases those with epilepsy themselves may not have known; if they only experienced what we now call simple seizures or absence attacks, then they probably never saw a doctor and were never diagnosed.

The scientific understanding of epilepsy developed in the nineteenth century with the work of Jackson and Gowers in the UK, and in the early twentieth century with the work of Erickson and Penfield in North America. However, these advances had little impact on most patients' care. In 1948, with the introduction of the National Health Service and the development of neurological services, epilepsy was more widely accepted as a neurological condition and medication became available. Nevertheless, there was still much to learn, and it was thought that epilepsy might be the cause of learning disability. There was no standard classification of epilepsy types or seizures, and many myths still surrounded this condition. Although medical services within the United Kingdom moved rapidly after the introduction of the Health Service, epilepsy services did not maintain the same pace.

REPORTS ON EPILEPSY SERVICES

In 1969 the Reid report was published; this was followed by the Bennett report in 1980 and 1982 (although this was never published in full), and a DHSS report in 1983, published in 1986. Comments made in these included:

> There should be postgraduate medical training and training for nurses.
>
> > (Reid, 1969)

> There is a lack of advice and counselling.
>
> Patients may experience difficulty getting information about their diagnosis.
>
> > (DHSS, 1983)

Other problems commented on included:

- The length of waiting lists

- Inadequate and irregular follow-up
- Lack of continuity of care
- Lack of attention to social requirements.

Some recommendations were that:

- There was a need for better training for both medical and nursing staff
- GPs were to be responsible for initial recognition of suspected epilepsy and referral to hospital
- District General hospitals were to be responsible for investigation, diagnosis and initiation of treatment
- Most patients should be followed up by GPs
- Patients with problematic epilepsy should be followed up by experts situated in a number of centres throughout the country.

Although the initial reports were undertaken on services provided to people with epilepsy and learning difficulties, later reports included a more widespread population.

In 1993, a document called *The Epilepsy Needs* was commissioned to investigate current services and how previous recommendations had been implemented. Compared to its predecessors, this was a brief report. A summary of the findings identified that in most areas little had changed, services were very patchy and fragmented, waiting lists were still long, there was no consistency in standards, and staff education was very limited. In the few areas where progress had been made, this was usually because of the drive of either an individual who was fortunate to be in a position of influence, or a small group who developed a service within a service to try and improve standards locally. There had been no national standards set, and no directives from any government about the implementation of changes recommended. An executive letter, EL95, also had little impact on changing services. A follow-up to *The Epilepsy Needs Document* was published in 1998: *Epilepsy Needs Revisited: A Revised Epilepsy Needs Document for the UK* (Brown *et al.*, 1998). This provides more recent information on epidemiology, and looks at advances in treatment and trends in health care, including the increasing number of specialist nurses and their role. It does not make any reference to whether these trends are national or whether they remain patchy.

The Clinical Standards Advisory Group

In 1998, a Clinical Standards Advisory Group (CSAG) was also commissioned to look at epilepsy services. This group undertook to investigate not only the service provided by sending questionnaires to health authorities, but also the patients' perception of the service. The report was completed in 1999 and published in March 2000, and a summary or its findings included the following:

- There was a lack of focus for services for people with epilepsy, and a lack of co-ordination between primary and secondary care
- Most patients seemed to be satisfied with their care, but felt that there was not enough contact between hospital and GP for effective monitoring
- Patients were concerned about lack of continuity and poor communication with their hospital care, but expressed satisfaction with specialist epilepsy services
- GPs were happy to manage day-to-day care and medication, but wanted support from specialists.

The report found that:
> ... there are still no well-defined parameters of health outcome measures that can be used nationally for the purpose of assessing health trends in epilepsy, equity of healthcare provision or efficacy of health policy ... Except on mortality there are no provisions for national audits to be undertaken.

The CSAG felt that:

- Changes should improve access and the equity of access
- The service should be more responsive and appropriate to patients needs
- There should be parallel goals of strengthening primary care and increasing specialization at the secondary care level.

These measures should:

- Improve the quality of care
- Improve medical outcomes
- Lessen the social exclusion and disability of people with epilepsy.

This report made recommendations aimed at creating an effective service that reflected patients' concerns. The CSAG felt that the changes recommended in the report could be implemented with local and regional provisions, and the laying down of clinical standards.

Local provisions

CSAG recommendations included the introduction of epilepsy centres throughout the UK to provide services for adults and children. These centres should be secondary-care focused, and:

- Provide dedicated adult and paediatric clinics
- Provide adult services to a population of 500 000 adults, and paediatric units to 200 000 children.

The CSAG also stated that: 'There will need to be an increase in the provision of epilepsy specialist nurses to support Epilepsy Centres'.

Regional provisions

The CSAG felt that NHS Executive Offices should be established to oversee, co-ordinate and monitor the setting up of epilepsy centres and paediatric clinics, and that these offices should:

- Assist in the development of tertiary services through Regional Specialist Commissioning Groups
- Ensure that there is adequate training available for medical personnel (e.g. establishing pre- and post-CCST fellowships), and make provision for training professionals allied to medicine (PAMs) (e.g. EEG technicians) and specialist nurses.

The CSAG also stated that: 'A national group should be established to evaluate performance and audit from a nationwide perspective'.

Clinical standards

The CSAG made the following recommendations:

1. NHS services should, at all levels, be more receptive to the views of patients and carers, and account for the needs of special groups (children, people with learning disability, women and the elderly). These needs could be incorporated into services provided by the epilepsy centres.
2. NHS services should provide equitable and easy access, effective communication, support and information.
3. Primary care should be strengthened by:
   - appointing a lead GP within a group practice to take the lead for improving the practice's service
   - ensuring greater clarity of the role of the GP vis-a-vis hospital services
   - introducing a better system of communication at the interface with secondary/tertiary care.
4. High standards of care for people with learning disabilities should be ensured by greater collaboration between specialist services (this could be done within epilepsy centres).
5. Adequate training should be provided for staff in A&E departments, protocols established for dealing with emergencies, and better lines of referral and communication ensured.
6. Neurosurgery for epilepsy should be available for all suitable patients in all areas of the UK:
   - referrals should be improved through epilepsy centres and paediatric clinics
   - patients should be assessed for suitability in units with appropriate facilities and adequate throughput and experience
   - surgical units should have necessary training, experience and throughput for a high quality of epilepsy surgery.
7. Patients with complex epilepsy (about 10 per cent of all patients) should have access to specialist facilities on a regional and supra-regional basis. These should include access to:
   - specialist investigations
   - neurosurgery
   - neuropsychiatry
   - inpatient care

- specialist assessment units
- second opinion where necessary.

The CSAG concluded by recommending that:

> … research into the effectiveness and value of epilepsy services, in particular of the changes recommended in the report, must be performed. Better systems for audit and the outcome data collection are needed to support service development.

Resource implications of the recommendations

The resource implications of the recommendations included the following:

CSAG comment that:-

1. A great deal can be done by reconfiguration of excising facilities.
2. Extra cost will depend on existing resources.
3. The marginal cost of running an epilepsy centre will include:
   - four consultant sessions
   - a full-time epilepsy specialist nurse
   - administration costs.
4. The cost of a paediatric clinic will include:
   - paediatric consultant sessions
   - a full-time epilepsy specialist nurse
   - administration costs.
5. Increased expenditure could include:
   - expansion or development of neurosurgical services
   - training for medical, nursing and PAMs, including in-house training
   - increasing audit and research activity.

Government response

The government's response to this report was that the principles and standards of good practice being put forward need to be tested for appropriateness at local level. It did not make any directive, and again left the standard of care available dependent on the patients' postcode. Again the problem of fragmented, patchy and sub-optimal care has been highlighted, but the political will to impose the implementation of the changes recommended is lacking. This contrasts sharply with the efforts being made for cardiac and cancer patients. Perhaps a stigmatized disease like epilepsy has less political appeal than these others, or perhaps the lobbying by the patient representative groups for cancer and heart have been more effective.

Neurological expertise

Parallel with the recognition of the needs of patients with epilepsy has been a geographic change in the distribution in expertise about the condition. At the end of the nineteenth century, neurological expertise was concentrated in London. By the latter half of the twentieth century, neurological expertise was concentrated in major teaching hospitals across the country. Over the last 20 years neurological services have become available in most district general hospitals, and in the last 10 years, with the development of the epilepsy specialist nurses, that expertise has been spreading into the community. Over the next 10 years, with the development of primary care services, it is important that knowledge about epilepsy is disseminated within the primary care team and particularly the practice nurses who are taking on an increasingly pivotal role within the NHS. Within a primary care group/trust it would make sense for some nurses to specialize in an area of expertise, and epilepsy is a prime candidate for that approach.

Not all nurses need to become experts, but if their knowledge and understanding are increased, and they are aware of where specialist advice exists locally, then the service provided will have a better chance of becoming more standardized nationally.

3

Implications for lifestyle

INTRODUCTION

In this chapter we will be discussing the impact of epilepsy on everyday living both for the person with epilepsy and for his or her carers.

The diagnosis of epilepsy often has major social and economic consequences for the person who receives the diagnosis. The label 'epileptic' results in the loss of freedoms most of us take for granted. For many people it is the effect that epilepsy will have on their lifestyle that is a major factor in coming to terms with the diagnosis. For some it is the feeling that this means loss of control and loss of independence. In addition, there is the uncertainty of how quickly, if ever, the seizures will be controlled. Their own attitude or fear of the word 'epilepsy' in the past will also influence their ability to cope now that they have the condition. If the correct support, advice and information can be given as early as possible, then they may find that they are more able to cope. This support will also be essential to the family carers. Their concerns will differ from those of the person with epilepsy, but will have a major influence on the level of overprotection that may occur.

One patient may be having one seizure a month and be holding down a job, bringing up a family, playing an active role in the local community and enjoying life. Another patient may be having one seizure a month and be unemployed, having marital difficulties and have withdrawn from society into a personal shell of misery. Can health care professionals help patients choose the more productive path? We believe they can.

It is in this area of support and giving information that nurses may be best placed to act because of their recognized role of educators and information givers. Often nurses are perceived by patients and relatives as having more time and being more approachable than the medical staff. The importance of the nurse in an outpatient setting is becoming increasingly pivotal as the emphasis of care is moving away from the traditional medical model with its preoccupation with diagnosis and medication.

The nurse does not have to be a specialist in this field of care to be able to make a difference. We have already discussed that because of the high incidence of epilepsy in the community, most nurses will have some contact with people with epilepsy. This means that we can all help, but it will be the degree of help that will differ. In some cases this will involve listening to the person's problems and knowing where to obtain the necessary advice or help. This can often be as important as being able to provide the information yourself. In Chapter 4 we will discuss in more detail the different ways in which different members of the nursing profession can become involved in improving the care and support available to people with epilepsy.

It is also true that most people with epilepsy in the UK will have little contact with specialist epilepsy services. Epilepsy is such a common problem that the responsibility for supporting people with epilepsy will fall on all health care professions, and particularly on nurses.

Here we will try to provide some basic factual information on what are thought to be the areas of advice most commonly requested or felt to be most important. These include education, employment, driving, safety in the home, holiday advice, and sport and leisure activities. Contraception and pregnancy will be covered in Chapter 9.

EPILEPSY AND EDUCATION

When talking about education we generally think about children and schooling, but we also need to think about students in higher education and mature students. The impact on all of these groups will present some common problems but will also raise different issues.

There are three main reasons why having epilepsy will have an impact on education: the seizures, the medication, and the ability to cope. In addition, consideration has to be given to the aim of education and how those aims may need modification in the light of a diagnosis of epilepsy. For example, if someone were studying to become an airline pilot when a diagnosis of epilepsy was made this would no longer be possible, and there would have to be some redirecting of educational aims.

In the following lists the main emphasis is on the child and education, although many of these factors also affect adults undertaking higher education.

Impact of the seizures on education

Seizures may impact on education in the following ways:

- Student absences from the classroom or school due to seizures during the day
- Students not attending school because of nocturnal seizures
- Students missing brief sections of lessons because of absences/seizures
- Poor memory and concentration due to tiredness from nocturnal seizures
- Autistic tendencies due to seizure activity/seizure type
- Bullying of the child with epilepsy because of 'being different'
- Bullying by the child with epilepsy as a defence mechanism-fear of the misunderstood
- Cognitive impairment from ongoing seizure activity.

All of these issues may lead to students not reaching their full potential educationally. This can mean a restricted choice of further education or employment, or problems in gaining any employment in the future.

Impact of the drug therapy on education

Drug therapy may impact on education in the following ways:

- Impaired cognitive function due to side effects
- Increased tiredness due to side effects
- Poor seizure control due to poor compliance or problems with medication
- Lack of understanding of drugs leading to poor compliance or incorrect dosing regime.

Reasons for underachieving

Some of the reasons for this underachieving include:

- Missed schooling or missed opportunities
- Lack of resources within the school, so lack of supervision in some lessons, e.g. home economics, science and sports
- Inappropriate advice about future prospects because of the advisor's lack of knowledge of epilepsy and its impact on employment
- Inappropriately reduced expectations on the part of educators.

Helping to avoid these problems

The way in which help within the school can be provided to prevent these problems arising will vary depending on the person's age, seizure type, and whether there are any associated medical problems.

The level of input will also vary depending on the knowledge of the professional involved regarding the condition. The important factor is that a potential problem should be recognized early, and help and support made available to patient, carers and teachers.

Areas to concentrate on include:

1. Identifying a child with epilepsy in a class.
2. Co-operation between the family and teachers to establish a protocol for action to be taken if the child has a seizure in the classroom, before this happens.
3. Providing advice for the teachers about dealing with the child's particular seizure type.
4. Advising the teachers about ways of ensuring that the child misses as little education as possible:
   - establish buddy systems within the class to provide help with work that may have been missed
   - provide instructions about homework in writing (a homework dairy to be used by teachers, child and parents) to ensure that instructions have not been missed due to absence seizures

- ensure that the child is reminded to check the homework diary each night.
5. Explaining that a child who may seem to be inattentive and daydreaming may be having a seizure.
6. Explaining that the child may be drowsy and having problems concentrating because of the medication.
7. Explaining that if the child's medication is being changed this may cause additional problems.
8. Ensuring that the teaching staff understand that it is important to inform the parents about any changes in the child's level of achievement or ability to concentrate – this may help in identifying problems early.
9. Reducing teacher anxiety and misconceptions.

Teachers can alert the health care system to educational problems that may be amenable to modification of medication. Remember that these are ordinary children who have a medical problem; as far as possible they should be treated in the same way as the other children in the class. The epilepsy needs to be taken into consideration, but should not be a reason for the child being excluded from any school activities.

EPILEPSY AND EMPLOYMENT

There are about 100 000 people with epilepsy at work in the United Kingdom. There is no evidence that people with epilepsy have higher sickness records or are less reliable than other employers. These facts, together with the right kinds of skills and self-confidence, are positive selling points to an employer.

These positive comments do not, however, make finding employment for people with epilepsy easy. In a survey undertaken in 1991 by Elwes and colleagues, the unemployment rate of people with epilepsy was found to be approximately 46 per cent compared with 19 per cent in an appropriately age- and sex-matched group. This discrepancy could not be related solely to the seizures. It therefore becomes more important to make sure that the correct qualifications are gained. Advice should be sought early to make sure that unrealistic aims for a chosen employment are not being set.

Even when employers are more understanding, the number of candidates for any position is usually high. During the short-listing process, most employers are looking for any excuse to whittle the number of candidates down to a manageable number. It is important that the people with epilepsy understand that the reason they did not succeed in most cases is not their epilepsy, but rather because there was a better candidate. They should not stop trying, although they must ensure that they are being realistic in their applications in accordance with their qualifications. It is, however, our impression that a diagnosis of epilepsy is still used far too often as an inappropriate reason for not considering people for employment. Should people with epilepsy be up front about declaring the diagnosis on the application form and risk being rejected inappropriately, or should they not declare it and risk being fired at a later date for not being honest? This is a difficult dilemma. A compromise may be to wait until they have an interview and can then explain in person. This is a question that nurses may be able to help patients resolve for themselves in their particular circumstances.

Employment restrictions

The employment open to people with epilepsy will usually depend on the type of seizure they experience, and the level of control of their seizures. Unfortunately there are some careers that will not be open to anyone who has had a seizure after the age of 5 years, even if they are seizure-free and not on medication. There are also some occupations in which employment may be difficult or dangerous, depending on the level of seizure control.

Dangerous occupations include those that involve working:

- At unprotected heights
- Near open water
- With high-voltage or open-circuit electricity
- With machinery that cannot be guarded
- Near chemicals
- On isolated sites
- On or near moving machinery.

Occupations where individual consideration would be given depending on the level of seizure control include:

- Teaching, depending on the subject
- Nursing
- Medicine
- The police force.

Some occupations are barred to those who have a history of seizures, even if well controlled. However, as regulations are constantly being updated it is always wise to contact the appropriate personnel or recruitment body to check the current recommendations.

Statutory barred occupations include:

- Airline or navigational pilot
- Army
- Navy
- Royal Air Force
- Coastguard (no specific regulations, but must have a high standard of fitness)
- Fire Brigade
- LGV/PCV driver
- Train driver.

It would be inappropriate for a people with epilepsy to apply for a position involving driving if they still have seizures of any sort, even simple partial seizures, as these prevent them from holding a driving licence.

The Disablement Employment Advisor at the Job Centre should be able to help with information about local employment and training courses available.

Discrimination

Any employer can be fined under the Employment Discrimination Act if it can be proved that a person was discriminated against and not employed on the grounds that he or she has epilepsy and if the epilepsy would not impair his or her ability to do the job. This may, however, be difficult to prove.

EPILEPSY AND DRIVING

The laws about driving with epilepsy are clearly defined in the manual *Medical Fitness to Drive* (DVLA, 1999). In this section we will briefly discuss the current information at the time of publication of this book.

What should you do?

1. Advise a person who has had a seizure to read the instructions on his or her driving licence.
2. The person concerned should inform the DVLA and the insurance company about the seizure/diagnosis. It is not sufficient to stop driving voluntarily and fail to notify the DVLA.
3. If you think that a patient is still driving but does not meet the requirements, depending on your role in the patient's care it may be appropriate to discuss your concerns with the patient, inform him or her of the law and document your concerns and actions.
4. If you are not sure of what action to take, then you should seek advice from the patient doctor, or the epilepsy specialist nurse if you have one locally.

Often discussing the potential implications of lack of insurance cover will have more of an impact than the advice about driving.

Seizure types imposing restrictions on driving

The following types of seizures impose restrictions on driving:

1. Tonic–clonic seizures, primary or secondary generalized.
2. Complex partial seizures.
3. Simple partial seizures with no loss of consciousness, including myoclonic jerks, motor seizure, 'auras' – *déjà vu*, olfactory, taste.
4. Provoked seizures. These are seizures with a definite trigger, and are non-recurring in a person with no history of epilepsy.

The trigger must be external and medically treatable. Driving is usually allowed when the underlying cause has been treated. Alcohol and illicit drugs do not qualify as triggers in these circumstances.

5. Single seizures. These are not regarded as epilepsy by the DVLA unless a continuing risk of seizures is demonstrated on EGG or a structural lesion on CT or MRI scanning. Driving is still prohibited for 1 year from the date of the seizure.

Statutory requirements regarding stopping driving

1. To hold an ordinary driving licence, a person should not drive for 1 year from the date of the last seizure. This rule applies whether there has been only one seizure and no medication has been started, or more than one and regular medication is used. It is important to know that a diagnosis of epilepsy does not have to be made for this law to apply.
2. If a person holds an ordinary licence and has only had nocturnal seizures (seizures during sleep) for a period of 3 years or more, he or she may be entitled to drive.
3. To hold a LGV/PCV licence, a person will have to have been free of seizures and off medication for a period of 10 years, and will also have to show that he or she does not have a continued increased risk of further seizures (e.g. a previous brain injury).

Non-statutory recommendations regarding stopping driving

Although the following are recommendations and not statutory requirements, the person must be advised about them. If the recommendations are not followed, there may be implications regarding insurance cover.

1. If a person has been seizure-free and is considering stopping medication, it is advised that he or she should not drive for the period of time that the medication is being reduced and for 6 months after it has been completely stopped.
2. If for some reason a person who is seizure-free is to remain

on medication but the drug needs to be changed, then it is also recommended that he or she should not drive while these changes are made (e.g. a female patient wishing to change drugs while planning a pregnancy).

> The onus of responsibility to inform the DVLA rests with the licence holder, not with the doctor or nurse. Anyone who continues to drive once the diagnosis of epilepsy has been made does so illegally until the above requirements are fulfilled. Car insurance, including third-party cover, is invalid if a person drives illegally.

Assistance available

While a person is unable to drive because of the diagnosis, some help is available:

- Rail passes are available for people with epilepsy; enquiries should be made to the local rail station.
- Recent changes in government guidelines mean that passes allowing assisted bus travel are now available; enquiries should be made at the local council offices.
- Other assistance may be available, including mobility allowance for people with multiple problems; enquiries should be made at the local Department of Social Services offices.

SAFETY IN THE HOME

Features to ensure a safe environment are important for everyone in every home. More people get injured in the home environment than at work. Where there is a member of the family with epilepsy, additional care may be needed to ensure that member's safety. It is important to remember that it is not the diagnosis of epilepsy that gives rise to additional problems, but the type of seizure and the level of control of the epilepsy. For a person who is seizure-free, there will be no additional risk. The risks are increased if the family member still has seizures, but will still vary depending on the type of seizure. A simple partial seizure with no loss of consciousness will carry little or no additional risk, whereas a complex partial seizure in which wandering may occur will cause problems. A generalized tonic–clonic seizure will cause increased risk of injury or even death. It is not the seizure itself that is usually the problem, but where it occurs and what the person is doing at the time.

The greatest dangers usually lie in the kitchen or the bathroom, although other areas of the house and surroundings do carry their own dangers. The most common problems are associated with electrical appliances, cooking and water. It is important to remember that although safety is of paramount importance, the need to maintain the person's independence and privacy must always be considered.

Listed below are some potential problem areas and ideas that may help to improve safety. Every person and situation will need to be judged individually; these are only suggestions that will need to be modified to meet these needs.

High-risk areas

Some potentially hazardous areas within the home where risk assessments may be needed include the following.

1. *The bath/shower room*: it is often recommended that showers are safer than baths for people with epilepsy; in most cases this is true, but you must consider the type of seizure and whether the person has any warning.
   - For people with any type of drop attack showers can be dangerous; having a seat and high controls in a shower may avoid some of these problems.
   - If there is only a bath, then make sure that only a small amount of water is used so that if a seizure occurs the person cannot slip below the water.
   - Whether a bath or shower is used, the person should not be alone in the house and the bathroom door must not be locked.
2. *The toilet area*:
   - Avoid small spaces at the side of the toilet where a person might become lodged on falling during a seizure.

3. *The kitchen*:
- Try to reduce the need to carry kettles or saucepans of boiling water
- If possible use a cooker guard
- When possible use a microwave if the seizures are poorly controlled.

4. *The stairs*:
- These can be a problem if a person wanders during a seizure. Ways of blocking the stair opening may need to be considered, although this may also present problems.

5. *The source of heating*:
- Use guards fixed to the wall around radiators and fires
- Enclose hot pipes.

6. *Furniture*:
- Reduce the number of small pieces of furniture
- Avoid glass in furniture (e.g. glass-topped tables)
- Avoid free standing lights
- Avoid trailing wires.

7. *The garden*:
- Remember that lawns are preferable to large paved areas
- Avoid pools and water gardens, which present a risk of drowning
- If the person wanders during a seizure, ensure that there is a secure gate.

All this may seem good advice, but it needs to be tempered with some common sense. Major household rebuilding would be unreasonable and perceived by the patient as silly advice if only a single seizure has occurred. The discussion should centre on sensible risk reduction that still allows the patient and family to function as near normally as possible.

HOLIDAY ADVICE

Having epilepsy should not prevent people from going on holiday if they want to. The type of holiday may vary depending on the needs of individuals, particularly if they have epilepsy in association with other medical problems. When arranging a holiday certain things will need to be taken into consideration, and it is best to inform the travel agent of the diagnosis at the time of booking if travelling abroad. The agent may be able to provide information about special provisions within hotels and local medical services if the epilepsy is not well controlled. There are hotels in England that provide for people with additional needs if necessary. There may be a local information office locally that could help.

Advice to a person with epilepsy who is arranging a holiday:

- Inform the travel agent about the epilepsy before booking, especially if the seizures are not controlled.
- Take out adequate insurance, checking that epilepsy is not excluded from the cover.
- Ask for the cost of insurance; the one suggested may be very expensive, and you may be able to get the same cover for less with someone else.
- Some airlines ask for a fitness to fly letter, ask the travel agent if they can check with the airline when you book. If not there is usually a contact number to ring when the tickets arrive.
- Take a copy of a current prescription with 'epilepsy' and the name of the drug clearly written on it. Remember that the drug may be available in other countries but may have a different name, so try to find out what it is called before travelling.
- Adjust the daily routine and times of the medication before travelling if there is going to be a large time difference when arriving and when returning home.
- Try to ensure that sleep deprivation is avoided where possible – get some rest on long flights because of the possible problems caused by lack of sleep.
- Take all medication in your hand luggage, and ensure that there is spare medication in your companion's hand luggage.
- Carry all medication in the original maker's packaging.
- Check with the doctor before having any vaccinations or malaria tablets.

First aid during seizures

Advice regarding the actions to be taken when a seizure occurs will need to be tailored to each individual's needs, and will vary depending on the length of time since diagnosis, the type of seizure, and whether the carers are professional or non-professional. As families learn to deal with the seizures, they will generally develop their own coping skills. They will usually need less support as time goes on; however, if the seizures prove difficult to control and the epilepsy is drug resistant, some families may need additional support and advice.

As with many other aspects of epilepsy, the first aid needed during a seizure depends on the seizure type.

Seizures requiring no intervention:
- Simple partial seizures with no loss of consciousness
- Complex partial seizures presenting as absence attacks
- Generalized absence seizures.

Seizures that may require intervention:
- Complex partial seizures where wandering may occur, to prevent injury
- Tonic or atonic seizures where injury has occurred.

Seizures where intervention will be required:
- Any seizure where injury has occurred
- Generalized seizures, whether primary or secondary generalized.

Individual advice will need to be given depending on the person's seizure type.

Basic information on dealing with different seizure types is given in Appendix 7.

SPORT AND LEISURE ACTIVITIES

It is not possible to cover advice on all sport and leisure activities, so in this section only general advice is given. Remember that this information is only about epilepsy, and any other problems that the person has must also be taken into consideration. When deciding whether or not epilepsy affects a person's ability to participate in any activity, many issues will need to be considered. The type of seizure will be a major factor.

Other points to consider include:

- If a seizure occurs while participating in the activity, will the person endanger anyone (including him or herself)?
- If so, how? Could the danger be avoided by ensuring that the person is not alone during the activity, by ensuring that there is someone around who knows what to do if a seizure occurs, or by performing the activity in different surroundings to improve safety?

It is important that people with epilepsy should be encouraged to participate in some type of sport or leisure activity within their capability. Sport and leisure activities are important not only for helping with general fitness, which will improve the person's well being, but also as a way for children to learn to develop social skills and relationships. If these skills are not developed, children may have problems in later life – their epilepsy may have become controlled, they may even be off their medication, but they may still be suffering from social problems related to the condition.

Some children will have difficulty in participating in any activities because of the type of seizures or the unwanted effects of medication. However, it is still important to encourage them to find some way of 'joining in' with others in play or sport. This will also help to assuage their feelings of 'being different'.

A significant factor will always be explanation to other people about epilepsy and the possible effects of the medication.

It is important to encourage adventure and sensible risk taking, as this will help to develop the skills practised in everyday life. We have a patient who rock climbs despite poorly controlled epilepsy. The risk is minimized by ensuring that the patient is properly roped to other climbers who have been trained to deal with seizures when they occur. They all feel that there is no more danger to the person with epilepsy than to any other member of the group. This may not be what you would advise, but if everyone knows the risks then they can make an informed choice.

> The advice in this chapter is meant to help the person with epilepsy and needs to be modified to the individual's needs. It should not be used to impose unnecessary restrictions.

4

The nurses role in epilepsy care

INTRODUCTION

This chapter is mainly aimed at nurses who are not specialists in the field of epilepsy. However, its contents may be of use to nurses working as specialists in the field as they set up links with their colleagues. Knowledge about the different roles of nurses in different areas allows for better team working. Specialist nurse roles will be defined by the nature of their post and the responsibilities outlined in their job description. In this chapter we will, however, cover nurse prescribing, which will be a particular issue for many specialist nurses.

Epilepsy has no boundaries of age, sex, race, colour or creed. The high incidence of the condition results in many patients having co-morbidity not directly associated with the epilepsy. There are numerous possible underlying causes that may result in the person developing epilepsy, and this means that a nurse in any branch of the profession may come into contact with a person with epilepsy.

We have already discussed the problems relating to the slow progress in addressing the stigma surrounding epilepsy and in improving epilepsy care, compared to conditions such as diabetes and asthma. In this chapter we will discuss potential ways in which nurses could make a difference in the way that this care is given in the future. The level of input will vary depending on the nursing post held and the nurse's individual knowledge of epilepsy. Some nurses may be involved in the patient's care in a way not associated with the epilepsy; in some situations the nurse may not even be aware that the person has epilepsy.

Making a Difference (DoH, 1999) is an NHS document outlining the government strategic intentions for nurses, midwives and health visitors within the new NHS. This document, presented in July 1999, includes recommendations on recruitment, education and training, modern career framework, improving working lives, professional self-regulation and strengthening leadership. It also includes setting standards for enhancing quality of care and working in new ways. This encourages nurses to work together to improve care and to play a full part in developing and implementing national service frameworks. Working together and sharing care are ways in which nurses can play an important part in advancing services and care for people with epilepsy.

There are a number of ways in which nurses can improve their input into patient care. The knowledge base to undertake this task is covered in the different chapters of this book. For all nurses, it is paramount that before undertaking new tasks they consider their own level of knowledge. In order to provide proper care a degree of competence based on knowledge is necessary. Nurses are accountable under the *Code of Professional Conduct* (UKCC, 1992a), and the *Scope of Professional Practice* (UKCC, 1992b). Other UKCC guidelines regarding good practice are *Standards for Records and Record Keeping* (UKCC, 1993) and *Clinical Governance* including benchmarking (Lugon and Secker-Walker, 1999). Clinical supervision can be a vital method of ensuring that good practice is followed and also providing peer support to colleagues. If this is undertaken correctly, it can help to form a basis for identifying and addressing training needs within a group.

Many nurses may feel that because of their current workload it is impractical to take on additional tasks. They could however play an integral role in improving care by being able to identify a problem and knowing how to obtain help, advice and support for the patient and carers.

NURSE PRESCRIBING FOR SPECIALIST NURSES

The Crown Report (DoH, 1999) contains new recommendations for nurses associated with the prescription, supply and administration of medicines. This outlines ways in which new groups of health care professionals with expertise in specific therapeutic areas may be able to prescribe prescription-only medicines.

The report lists the following options for nurse involvement in prescribing:

1. Maintaining the *status quo*
2. Prescribing from a limited formulary
3. Prescribing from the full formulary of general sales list and pharmacy medicines and prescription-only drugs (not controlled drugs).

The RCN wanted the government to consider including controlled drugs to give full prescribing rights.

This report discusses the possibility of two levels of prescribers:

1. Independent prescribers, responsible for assessing undiagnosed patients and with the authority to prescribe medicines. These may include family planning nurses, tissue viability nurses, chiropodists and podiatrists, specialist physiotherapists and optometrists.
2. Dependent prescribers, responsible for the continuing care of patients and with the authority to prescribe within clinical guidelines or to issue repeat prescriptions. These may include specialist diabetic nurses, specialist asthma nurses, specialist palliative care nurses, pharmacists in specialist areas, and pharmacists carrying out reviews of patients' medicines.

It also recommends that a UK advisory body assesses submissions from professional organizations for individuals to become independent or dependent prescribers, and states that newly authorized groups of prescribers should not normally be allowed to prescribe medicines in the following categories:

- Controlled drugs (drugs subject to the Misuse of Drugs Act 1971)
- Unlicensed drugs, or drugs used outside their licensed indications.

At present there has been limited implementation of this report. Some nurse practitioners will be able to prescribe in emergency situation where a patient group directive exists outlining the use of a specific drug. These patient group directives cover one-off changes of medication, usually in secondary care. A patient group directive needs to exist for each drug that may potentially be prescribed by the nurses nominated within a unit. There are no recommendations at present to cover nurses needing to make ongoing changes in patients' medication, or to initiate long-term medication change plans. At present nurses, including specialist nurses in the field of epilepsy care, are not covered by these new recommendations.

The British Medical Association (BMA) expressed concerns that even with additional training nurses would not be equipped to prescribe from the full formulary. They suggested that all general sales list items and pharmacy medicines be added to the nurse prescribing formulary, with a specific range of prescription-only drugs covering certain conditions being included. They seemed concerned that giving nurses additional training and allowing them to prescribe was turning them into doctors. The Royal College of General Practitioners (RCGP) responded that they felt that, with the correct training, support and agreed guidelines, these proposals could only benefit patient care.

The RCN does not feel that allowing nurses to prescribe is developing their role into that of a doctor. Specifically named nurses would be allowed to prescribe drugs used within their specialist field; they would not be allowed to prescribe generally. This would enhance their roles of providing care, advice and support and being the patients advocate, still leaving the doctors to investigate, diagnose and decide on overall methods of treatment. For many years nurses with experience in their particular area of care have advised some grades of medical staff about medication and then had to wait for the doctor to write the prescription.

NON-SPECIALIST NURSING INPUT INTO CARE OF PATIENTS WITH EPILEPSY

The following information is based on the North Staffordshire local shared care guidelines for ways in which practice nurses could be involved in monitoring patients with epilepsy in primary care. This template can be adapted to fit with a practice's established methods of monitoring patients. It could also be adapted for use by nurses working within other areas of primary care or in outpatient units within a hospital.

ESTABLISHING CRITERIA OF CARE FOR MONITORING PATIENTS WITH EPILEPSY

Initial contact following a generalized seizure may be with the GP or local A&E services. The diagnosis of epilepsy is usually made within secondary care.

Criteria for the monitoring of individual patients should be established between primary and secondary care when the diagnosis is made. The site for monitoring may change as the patient's condition progresses, depending on:

- The age of the patient at diagnosis
- The level of seizure control obtained
- The amount of medication needed
- Any changes in the patient's circumstances
- Whether there is co-morbidity.

The main objectives of monitoring should be:

- To improve patient care
- To improve patients' and carers' understanding of epilepsy
- To improve communication between the patient and primary/secondary care.

This should in turn:

- Improve seizure control
- Reduce unwanted drug profiles
- Improve patients' quality of life
- Reduce the social stigma associated with the condition.

MONITORING EPILEPSY IN PRIMARY CARE

A monitoring service could be established as a joint venture by a general practitioner and a practice nurse in clinic together, or as a practice nurse clinic that is overseen by a general practitioner. This protocol could also be adapted for district nurses visiting patients at home.

What could a practice nurse achieve by seeing patients with epilepsy?

Involvement by this practice nurse could be invaluable in co-ordinating the care of patients with co-morbidity, and thus helping to avoid the problem of conditions being treated in isolation. Often the practice nurse is the first point of contact for patients with chronic conditions, so there is no reason why epilepsy should be different.

The level of input into care by the nurse may vary from practice to practice. It may be that it is not felt appropriate for the practice nurse to be involved in the management of epilepsy, or there may not be a practice nurse.

How could improvement be achieved within the practice?

Improvement could be achieved with a nominated person (or persons) within the practice:

- Acting as a first point of contact for patients and carers (parameters to be agreed within each individual practice)
- Acting as a link between the practice and the epilepsy specialist nurse
- Acting as a link with school nurses, community midwife, CPN and RNMH.

Newly diagnosed patients and patients on medication with non-problematic epilepsy could also be reviewed.

The following models can be used either where there is an established practice-based epilepsy clinic, or where patients are seen as part of a daily appointment system. They can also be used if the patient needs to be seen at home. The criteria on which these models are based are those used within our nurse-led epilepsy clinic currently established within local secondary care. The models are based on primary care staff having access to a clinical nurse specialist in epilepsy for advice and support. The specialist nurse may be able to offer advice or obtain advice from the consultant, thereby speeding up the care process.

The use of these protocols should enable consistency of care and improved communication between primary and secondary care.

Newly diagnosed patients

Criteria for seeing the patient

Once the diagnosis has been established, the patient can be seen along with a member of the family who has witnessed a seizure. This will allow you to:

1. Obtain a written description of the seizure from the patient and the witness for surgery records. If one has been recorded previously by the GP, then check that this has not changed. Ensure that if the patient has more than one type of seizure, all types are recorded.
2. Record any medication being taken, whether a brand or generic drug, the dose, and the time of day that it is taken.
3. Ensure that the importance of drug compliance has been discussed with the patient.
4. Ensure that patients know that they are entitled to free prescriptions.
5. Ensure that the patient has a seizure diary card and is completing this.
6. Ensure that initial advice has been given as appropriate according to an agreed advice checklist. Record what advice the patient has been given (the person seeing the patient will not necessarily be expected to give advice but to establish any areas not covered and know where the patient can obtain any additional advice necessary).
7. Establish a method of contact with the patient and carer.
8. Establish whether the patient is to be reviewed by the epilepsy specialist nurse and arrange contact with the specialist nurse if necessary.
9. Arrange a review appointment with the patient.

Patients with non-problematic epilepsy

Criteria to be followed when seeing the patient

These patients can be seen annually to monitor progress, but may need to be seen more often if requested by the GP. This will allow you to:

1. Check the patient's diary card and record the seizure frequency in surgery notes:

- if the patient is seizure-free, then record the date of the last seizure
- ensure that this is done for all types of seizures.

2. Check the medication being taken and record it in the notes:
   - ask the patient what medication is being taken and at what time; this should then be checked against repeat prescriptions (don't forget to check the name of the drug – brand or generic; if this has changed from the last visit, query why and check if seizure control or any unwanted side effects have changed).

3. Check for any unwanted effects of the medication (e.g. drowsiness, double vision, rash).

4. Recheck the advice sheet to establish that no new advice is needed. The patient's circumstances may have changed.

5. Check with female patients regarding contraception (there are interactions between some anti-epileptic drugs and the combined oral contraceptive pill).

6. Remind female patients about the need for pre-pregnancy advice (e.g. the need to take folic acid 5 mg daily for at least 3 months prior to conception, and to be seen by a specialist for review of their medication).

7. Check that children have no problems at school related to their epilepsy.

8. Check if patients need advice about higher education or types of employment.

9. Arrange the next review appointment.

The aim of this process is to check the patient's status and to identify any possible problem areas. Remember that you do not need to know all of the answers; just where to obtain them or where to refer the patient for further screening or advice. This should have been established within the practice before you see any patients.

Potential problems and what should be done

If the monitoring is to be carried out by the practice nurse, then a protocol for seeing patients should be established before the clinic commences and documentation agreed for recording each visit. The main purpose is to be able to recognize problems and to follow the established protocols.

The main problem areas and possible ways of dealing with them include:

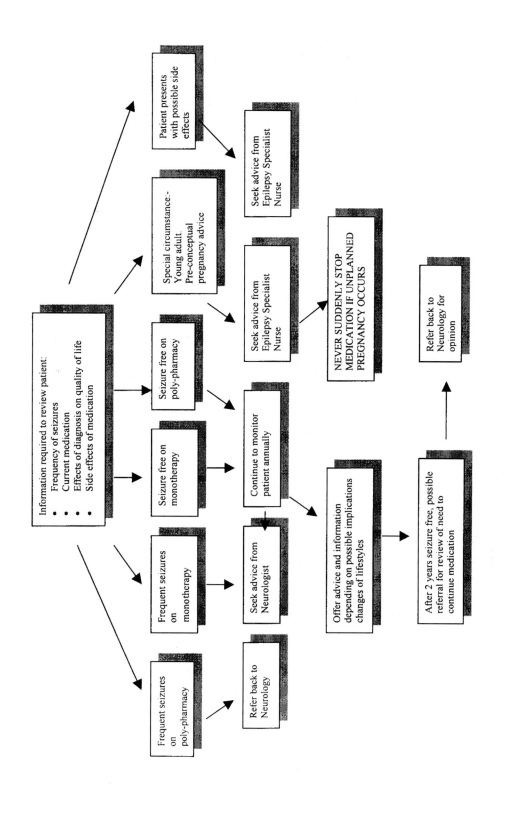

Figure 4.1 A suggested monitoring system for patients with a long-standing diagnosis of epilepsy.

1. Unwanted effects of the medication – seek advice from the GP or contact the specialist nurse. *Remember that monitoring drug levels is not usually the answer.* These levels are often only helpful in telling you that the patient has taken the medication; not how it is acting. For some patients there is a fine line between seizure control and the unwanted effects of the drugs, and some patients prefer the latter to having seizures. You may not always be helping by arranging for medication to be reduced.

2. A change in the patient's circumstances requiring new advice:
   - contraception
   - changing employment
   - going on holiday.

3. Female patients contemplating pregnancy – refer to the GP and/or the specialist nurse.

4. Female patients presenting with an unplanned pregnancy – check that medication has not been suddenly discontinued. Refer to the GP, and the specialist nurse if appropriate. *Remember that the medication should not be stopped suddenly in this situation.* This can be dangerous and will have little effect regarding the implications of drugs on the foetus. Any structural damage is usually done within the first 7–28 days following conception.

5. Patients querying withdrawal of medication – refer to the GP; these patients may need to be referred to a neurologist for advice about the risk of withdrawal.

Patients with problematic or intractable epilepsy

These patients should be under regular review by a consultant and the specialist nurse. The GP may still want the patient to be reviewed within the practice. This will help to establish that any changes recommended by secondary care are being undertaken, and help to improve communication.

PRIMARY CARE NURSES IN THE COMMUNITY

Midwives

Midwifery intervention can be undertaken by community and hospital midwives. Although seizure control and medication does not come into their remit of care, midwives can play an important part in ensuring that the woman is receiving advice and is being monitored appropriately. Specific information relating to epilepsy and pregnancy is given in Chapter 9.
Midwives can:

- Check whether the woman has taken folic acid 5 mg daily; in some cases this may be continued for the whole of the pregnancy
- Check the level of control of the epilepsy and the medication taken
- Check whether the woman is under the care of a neurologist and in contact with a specialist nurse
- Ensure that the woman will have a high-resolution scan at 20 weeks' gestation to check for foetal abnormalities
- Check whether the women will require vitamin K for last 4 weeks of the pregnancy because of her medication
- Check whether advice has been given about potential triggers for seizures during the delivery
- Try to ensure that the labour and delivery are not prolonged, as this is a potential cause of seizures during or immediately after delivery
- Check whether advice has been given about breast-feeding and safety when caring for the baby.

School nurses

The level of input will depend on the type of school covered by the nurse. Nurses attached to special schools where there may be a high incidence of epilepsy will be more involved with the medication and possibly with the administration of rectal diazepam. Nurses attached to mainstream schools may have little input into care, although they can play an important part in ensuring that the child's education is not disrupted by the epilepsy. For more information on children and epilepsy, see Chapter 8.

School nurses can:

- Ensure that he or she knows of any child in their school with epilepsy
- Check the level of seizure control
- Check whether medication is required at school
- Implement a policy of care to be followed if the child has a seizure in school.

They can help by:

- Ensuring that staff know how to deal with a seizure if one occurs
- Ensuring that the teachers understand the possible impact on the child's education of the epilepsy and the drugs
- Ensuring that the child is not excluded from lessons such as swimming, domestic science and CDT because of lack of understanding within the school.

Community learning disability nurses

Owing to the high incidence of epilepsy in people with learning disabilities, these nurses will usually have an increased level of knowledge of this condition. They can play an important part in establishing the difference between seizures and behavioural problems. This can avoid unnecessary changes in medication and the over-prescribing of anticonvulsant medication. They can also provide a link between home carers, GPs and hospital services to ensure that recommended changes are initiated correctly.

Health visitors

Although health visitors may not be directly involved in the care of people with epilepsy, they may be able to help support the family where there is an affected child. Where a health visitor is involved with the care of a pre-school child with epilepsy they can help by:

- Providing support to the family
- Obtaining information leaflets
- Trying to ensure that the child is not overprotected
- Trying to ensure that other children in the family are not affected by the problem.

Health visitors can also:

- Help in the monitoring and advice given to new mothers who have epilepsy about the safety aspect of childcare
- Act as a link to the GP and hospital services.

NURSING IN SECONDARY CARE

In this section we will provide examples of how nurses in secondary care can try to improve services and standards of care.

In most acute trust hospitals there will be a neurology service providing care for people with epilepsy. With the expansion of specialist nurse services since the early 1990s, many of these units will now have a specialist nurse. These specialist nurses will still only provide a service to a proportion of patients with epilepsy because of the incidence of the condition, and the service they provide will depend on the remit of their post. Most acute trust hospitals providing a service to a population of 250 000–500 000 will potentially have approximately 2500–5000 patients with epilepsy. Some hospitals may have specific units providing specialist epilepsy care.

For many nurses working within a secondary care setting their involvement will be on a short-term basis; because of this most secondary care nurses working outside the neurology services will not be able to establish monitoring systems as suggested for primary care. In some areas the epilepsy service is managed from a speciality other than neurology. As in primary care, the nurse may not be caring for patients as a direct result of a problem with their epilepsy. Nurses working on units outside neurology services where patients with epilepsy may be admitted should establish what services are available within their hospital. They should also establish whether there is a specialist nurse within their hospital, and what service and support they can obtain.

Within secondary care the nurse input could be divided into acute emergency care, short-term inpatient care and ongoing outpatient care.

Nurses in accident and emergency/medical assessment units

Nurses working within these areas will be caring for patients presenting with a first seizure, because of a prolonged or complicated seizure, or because of injury as a result of a seizure. Many of these patients will recover spontaneously from the seizure and not require admission, although some will have potentially life-threatening complications.

In this setting, nurses need to be aware of:

- The complications of tonic–clonic status epilepticus
- Complex partial seizures presenting as aggression or drug toxicity
- Problems with overuse of diazepam
- Patients with non-epileptic attack disorder potentially being wrongly treated with anti-epileptic drugs
- Patients presenting following a first seizure who are not admitted; these patients need to be advised about the driving regulations, and the family needs to be advised about what to do if a second seizure occurs.

Establishing contact with a specialist nurse within the hospital can help in the developing of protocols and referral guidelines between A&E and neurology services.

Ward nurses

Ward nurses' input will be direct nursing care depending on the patient's immediate needs. Their level of input may vary depending on the type of ward – neurological or general medical – and includes:

- Obtaining a seizure description
- Monitoring seizure frequency
- Administering medication

- Monitoring for side effects of medication
- Checking advice given to patients
- Arranging for referral to a specialist nurse if this is possible within the hospital
- Ensuring that the patient knows about potential problems with brand switching of drugs, and the importance of compliance and regular times of taking drugs
- Ensuring that the patient knows about free prescriptions
- Ensuring that the patient knows about driving regulations
- Checking that female patients know about problems with contraception and the need for pre-pregnancy advice.

Where patients are admitted because of problems other than their epilepsy, the ward nurse should:

- Ensure that the patient continues on his or her regular medication
- Contact the services providing care of the epilepsy if there are any problems with the epilepsy or if the patient requests that such services are advised of the admission.

Intensive care nurses

In this situation the care will be the direct monitoring of the patient's critical situation. If there is a specialist nurse based at the hospital, he or she may be able to help support the family and provide a link between anaesthetic and neurological medical staff.

Nurses on neurology/medical outpatient clinics

Where there is a specialist nurse service available, some patients with epilepsy will be monitored within this service. For the patients who are not seen within the specialist nurse service, other nurses (link nurses) within the clinic could help to provide additional support to the patients and to the specialist nurse. Few services have the luxury of being able to provide specialist epilepsy nurse cover for 24 hours a day, 7 days a week, 52 weeks a year, so having other nurses who have some specialist knowledge and can link in with the specialist nurse when he or she is available is invaluable.

If there is no specialist nurse service, then monitoring could be undertaken by a nominated nurse or nurses within the out patient unit following the protocol suggested for primary care. This should be done in conjunction with the medical staff leading the epilepsy care within the unit. If patients with epilepsy are seen within general medical clinics by different consultants, a clinic nurse helping to provide a monitoring service could help to improve and standardize care.

CONCLUSION

It is hoped that by using and adapting the information within this chapter, nurses in all branches of the profession can become involved in helping to improve epilepsy care.

You can help by:

- Knowing what epilepsy services are available locally
- Establishing links with your local specialist service if there is one
- Knowing where to obtain help, advice and information for your patients if there is no local specialist service
- Developing links with other local service providers
- Helping to develop monitoring services within your workplace.

If you are not able to establish a formal monitoring service, then even a small change in your practice may make a big difference to a person with epilepsy.

5 The biochemical basis of epilepsy

INTRODUCTION

In general, having an understanding of the biochemical basis of epilepsy is not essential to being involved in the patient's care. However, as some of the drug therapies are now being designed to target specific parts of the biochemical system, having some understanding of the chemistry can be useful. One of the questions patients ask is, 'Why me?'. It may be impossible to give a full answer to this question, but having some understanding of the underlying biochemistry may at times be helpful in explaining what causes a seizure to occur.

NEURONES ARE INTRINSICALLY UNSTABLE

For the brain or any nervous system to work, neurones (Figure 5.1) have to fire off, or depolarize. There is a potential difference of about 70 mV between the inside of a cell and the outside. This electrical potential is like the voltage difference between the two

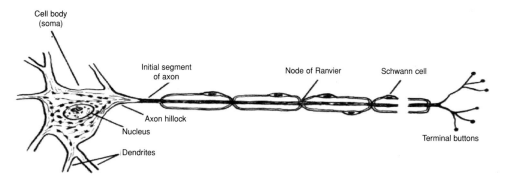

Figure 5.1 Anatomy of a neurone.

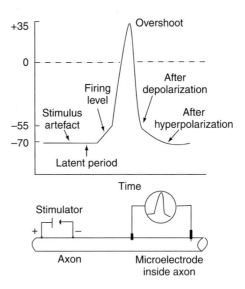

Figure 5.2 Depolarization of an axon.

ends of a battery. The battery has chemicals in it to maintain its electrical potential, and so does the cell; inside is potassium, and outside is sodium. The sodium would normally diffuse into the cell, down the concentration gradient, but it cannot because the cell membrane forms a barrier. This results in sodium ions (Na^+) being held on the outside, making the outside of the cell positive relative to the negative inside. If holes open in the cell membrane, then sodium ions (Na^+) will rush through the channel, causing the cell membrane potential difference to move closer to neutral (Figure 5.2).

These channels are gated; they only open under certain circumstances. Some channels are gated by chemicals (neurotransmitters) and some by the voltage potential across them (voltage-gated channels; Figure 5.3). The gates are automatically closed after a time, allowing the cell's potential to be restored – repolarization. These discharges can be transmitted by the neurone to a neighbouring neurone along an axon. At the end of the axon, an excitatory neurotransmitter such as acetylcholine may be released. If this occurs, it will open chemically-gated channels, allowing depolarization of the next cell. If sufficient depolarization occurs, then the next neurone's voltage-gated channels will fire off and that neurone will depolarize and pass its message to the next neurone. While the neurone is firing it is

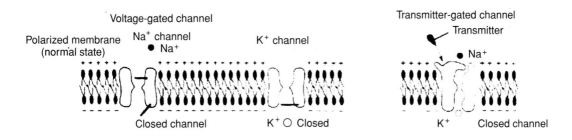

Figure 5.3 Voltage-gated and transmitter-gated channels.

know as excited, able to pass on messages; it then becomes inhibited, less able to pass messages.

Glutamate and asparate are the two major excitatory neurotransmitters in the CNS. They cause neurones to depolarize (fire off), and are involved in the initiation and spread of seizures. There are three major post-synaptic glutamate receptor types: AMPA, quiaqualate and NMDA. They are named after the chemicals to which they preferentially bind. While NMDA antagonists theoretically seem to be potentially attractive anti-epileptic drugs (AEDs), these substances tend to produce unacceptable psychological side effects.

GABA is the major inhibitory neurotransmitter in the central nervous system (CNS), in that it reduces the chances of a neurone firing off. This activity reduces the likelihood of a seizure occurring. GABA is synthesized from glutamic acid by decarboxylation within the brain. The GABA receptor allows the outlet of chloride ions from the cell, resulting in hyperpolarization, taking the cell membrane potential further away from its threshold (the point at which it will fire off). The GABA receptor has benzodiazapine and barbiturate receptor sites in close proximity, which enhance the activity of the receptors.

WHY DO SEIZURES OCCUR?

Seizures occur as a result of a disruption in the normal firing and resting patterns of the neurone. There may be a collection of damaged neurones, or a chemical disruption may occur. The lack of control may be due to over-activity of the excitatory neurotransmitters, or under-activity of the inhibitory neurotransmitters. Either of these actions will cause over-firing of a group of neurones, and the increased electrical activity produced results in the seizure. These changes may occur in a small area of the brain, causing a partial seizure, or may spread throughout the cortex, causing a generalized seizure.

Most seizures are 'self limiting' – that is, they will spontaneously resolve. The reason for this is not fully understood. This may be because of a naturally increasing release of inhibitory neurotransmitters.

HOW DO ANTI-EPILEPTIC DRUGS WORK?

In most cases the mode of action of these drugs is not fully understood, although there is some understanding of which part of the action potential is affected by the drug:

- Carbamazepine acts on the sodium channel conductance, also on the NMDA receptors.
- Gabapentin was designed as a GABA analogue, but does not bind at known GABAminergic sites, yet still has an anti-epileptic effect. Its action is not certain, but it is thought to act on calcium channels.
- Lamotrigine inhibits the release of glutamates and blocks sodium conduction.
- Valproate increases the synthesis and decreases the breakdown of GABA.
- Vigabatrin is a suicidal inhibitor of GABA transaminase, which is involved in its breakdown.
- Phenytoin blocks sodium channels and acts on voltage-dependant neurotransmission.
- Topiramate is supposed to have three sites of action: it reduces epileptic discharges from voltage-sensitive sodium channels; it enhances GABA at the receptor; and it antagonizes the AMPA glutamate receptors.

What can you tell patients?

- That you may not know the cause of their epilepsy
- Even where there is an underlying lesion that may be related, you cannot say why they developed epilepsy when someone else with a similar lesion may not do so
- You cannot say when a seizure may occur, although sometimes a potential trigger may be identified
- You cannot say exactly how the drugs work, but they have an effect on helping to stabilize the chemicals that control the electrical activity in the brain
- The doctor will try to control their epilepsy with one drug, although this may not be possible – because there is more than one chemical reaction controlling the electrical activity, some patients may need a combination of drugs to control their epilepsy
- The drugs need to be taken daily and at regular intervals to help obtain the best control of their epilepsy.

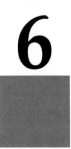

6

Making the diagnosis, investigations and classification of seizures

INTRODUCTION

The diagnosis of epilepsy is clinical. This means that the history obtained from the patient and any observers is the most important factor in making the diagnosis. This information will help to determine any possible underlying cause, and will be important in aiding the diagnosis of some seizure types and syndromes. The history may reveal other possible causes for the episodes of loss of consciousness than epilepsy. This will be of great importance in helping to determine treatment type, prognosis outcomes, and support needed, to ensure the best possible outcome. There is nothing like making an incorrect diagnosis to mess up a patient's management!

Although there are now many sophisticated forms of investigation available to aid diagnosis, the most important factor in the diagnosis of epilepsy still remains the history of events from the person who had the episode, and from an eyewitness. It is these that will form the basis for this section.

It is appropriate that any patient suspected of having epilepsy should be referred to a neurologist or epilepsy specialist, because of the complexity of making the diagnosis. However, there are important factors that can be considered by the GP or primary care nurse. The better the initial information obtained and the more accurate the description of events, as near to the time of occurrence as possible, the better the chance of a correct diagnosis.

When a patient presents with a single seizure, an accurate description needs to be well documented. This will enable any subsequent events to be compared for similarities. Any comparison will not then be reliant on people's memories.

When referrals are made, as much information as possible should be included. Parents or families should be advised to take a written description of the attack to the clinic. This is essential, especially if the person who witnessed the attack cannot attend the clinic (e.g. a school teacher or child minder).

INFORMATION NEEDED TO HELP IN MAKING THE DIAGNOSIS

There follows a suggested procedure for when a patient presents with a seizure.

1. Obtain a detailed step-by-step description of the subjective experience of the attack from the patient, including the post-ictal period.
2. Obtain a detailed step-by-step description of the attack as witnessed by an observer.
3. Establish the patient's present medical history to determine:
   • any possible trigger factors, e.g. lack of sleep/alcohol/ drugs
   • any underlying structural cause, e.g. tumour/infarction
   • any inflammatory or metabolic problems.
4. Establish the patient's past medical history to identify any possible relevant factors:
   • neonatal history/febrile convulsions/head injuries.
5. If this was the first generalized tonic–clonic seizure, try to establish whether the person has ever experienced any episodes that could have been partial or complex partial seizures. Is there any evidence of myoclonus that has not previously been identified?
6. Investigate the possibility of any underlying cause, but remember that only 30–40 per cent of cases of epilepsy will have such identifiable underlying cause.
7. Undertake a neurological and general medical examination to determine general health.

Co-morbidity

Possible underlying causes to consider include:

• Cerebral tumour

- Cerebral infections
- Cerebrovascular events
- Trauma
- Congenital abnormalities.

Some of these will require urgent specialist treatment, not all of them are life threatening, and some will require no intervention. However, identifying an underlying cause may help in determining the most appropriate treatment and prognosis. Often patients and their relatives need to be reassured that there is no serious brain illness causing the epilepsy.

Some groups of patients have an increased incidence of epilepsy compared to the general population (Table 6.1). This is possibly because the condition may lower an individual's seizure threshold and therefore increase the risk of them developing epilepsy.

Table 6.1 Conditions that increase an individual's risk of developing epilepsy

Condition	Risk of epilepsy
Stroke	Occurs in approximately 10%
Multiple sclerosis	Risk is increased by approximately 1–5%
Alzheimer's disease	Occurs in approximately 33%
Huntingdon's chorea	Occurs in approximately 5%
Wilson's disease	Occurs in approximately 6%
Creutzfelt–Jakob disease	Occurs in approximately 10%
Systemic lupus erythematosis	Increased risk

Drugs used for the treatment of some medical conditions may lower seizure thresholds. This may result in the onset of epilepsy or loss of control in people with an established diagnosis. These include:

- Diabetes
- Depression
- Cardiac dysrhythmias
- Alcohol withdrawal
- Malaria
- Hormonal therapy
- Anaesthetics

A list of potentially epileptogenic drugs is included in Chapter 7. Recreational drug usage may also trigger seizures.

Taking a history of the episode

You will need:

1. A description of the episode from the patient.
2. An eye-witness account.

You may wish to use a reminder of the information needed. The one in the box was designed for our local unit, and has also been adopted for use in some learning disability care homes.

Seizure description information sheet

The purpose of this information is to provide as clear a statement as possible of what happened before, during and after an attack. This should include what the eye witness observed and also where possible/as soon as possible information from the patient regarding what they recall of events prior to, during and after the attack. You should include the following information where possible.

Eye-witness account

1. What was the person doing at the time of onset?
2. Was there any change in behaviour?
3. Had the person just fallen asleep or woken up?
4. What called your attention to the attack – a cry or shout?
5. Did the attack start in one part of the body (e.g. head turning to one side, slurred speech)?
6. Did the attack progress to involve other parts of the body (e.g. one side, all limbs)?
7. How did the attack progress (e.g. slowly, quickly)?
8. Did the person become stiff and then fall?
9. Did the person suddenly become floppy and then fall?
10. Was there shaking of any part of the body?
11. Was one side of the body affected more then the other?
12. Was the person able to respond?

13. Was there any loss of consciousness, altered awareness, or state of confusion?
14. Was there any change in breathing pattern or change in skin colour (e.g. flushed, cyanosis)?
15. Did the person talk or perform any actions during the attack?
16. Was there any incontinence during the attack?
17. Where there any injuries as a result of the attack?
18. How did the person behave after the attack (e.g. alert, drowsy, confused)?
19. How long did the person take to recover fully from the attack?
20. What did the person remember about the attack, before, during and after it happened?
21. How long did each part of the attack last?

Patient's account
1. How did the patient feel prior to the attack?
2. What does the patient remember prior to the attack?
3. Can the patient remember the onset?
4. Does the patient remember anything during the episode?
5. What does the patient remember after the episode?
6. How did the patient feel after the episode?

Please remember that it is important to give as much information as possible. You will help the doctor to reach the correct diagnosis, and therefore help in the decision towards the correct line of treatment.

Differential diagnosis

There is a wide differential diagnosis to consider when a patient presents with seizures. In reality it is not as daunting as Table 6.2 suggests, and a bit of common sense and a good listening ear will rapidly direct you to the correct diagnosis most of the time.

Table 6.2 Differential diagnosis

	Adult	Child
Syncope	Postural hypotension	Simple faints
	Vaso-vagal episodes	Vaso-vagal episodes
Cerebrovascular	Transient ischaemic episodes	Benign paroxysmal vertigo
Cardiac	Heart block	Reflex bradycardia (anoxic seizures)
	Arrhythmia	Arrhythmia
Behavioural	Hyperventilation	Hyperventilation
		Breath-holding
	Temper tantrums	Temper tantrums
	Rocking	Rocking
		Head-banging
		Daydreaming
	Tics	Tics
	Panic attack	Panic attack
	Munchausen's syndrome/	Munchausen's syndrome/
	Munchausen by proxy	Munchausen by proxy
Other causes	Migraine	Migraine
	Narcolepsy and cataplexy	
	Hypoglycaemic episodes	Hypoglycaemic episodes
	Night terrors	Night terrors
		Nightmares
	Sleep walking	Sleep walking
		Benign neonatal, infantile or sleep myoclonus
		Febrile convulsions
	Alcohol/drug-induced seizures	Alcohol/drug-induced seizures
	Metabolic seizures	Metabolic seizures

Helping to differentiate

In epilepsy:
- There is abruptness of onset, usually with no warning
- There is loss of awareness
- The length of the attack may vary
- The attacks are stereotyped
- Recovery is usually followed by a period of confusion
- The attack is often followed by a period of sleepiness/ headache

- The attacks recur spontaneously
- A trigger factor is not usually identified (Table 6.3).

In syncope or cardiovascular disease:
- Attacks are usually slower in onset
- Loss of consciousness is often preceded by symptoms of light-headedness and a feeling of things becoming distant/greying out of vision
- Recovery is usually quick
- The attack can usually be aborted by the person lying down at the onset of symptoms
- There is no period of confusion or sleepiness after the episode
- A trigger factor is often identifiable – e.g. heat, posture, over-crowded room.

On some occasions syncope may be accompanied by twitching and even urinary incontinence, so leading to misdiagnosis (see Table 6.3).

Table 6.3 Differentiating between epilepsy and syncope

Observation	Seizure	Syncope
Posture	Any position	Upright
Pallor and sweating	Uncommon	Usually present
Onset	Sudden/with aura	Gradual
Injury	Not uncommon	Rare
Convulsive jerking	Common	Not uncommon
Incontinence	Common	May occur
Unconsciousness	May last for minutes	Lasts seconds
Recovery	Often slow	Rapid
Post-episode confusion	Common	Rare
Frequency	May be frequent	Rare
Precipitating factors	• Lack of sleep • Alcohol • Menstruation • Stress • Photosensitivity	• Crowded places • Lack of food • Pain

In hypoglycaemia:

- The attack is usually gradual in onset
- The person may look vacant, be confused and have slurred speech
- Some trembling may be observed
- There is sweating and palpitation
- There will be loss of consciousness if not treated
- There may be confusion as consciousness returns after the administration of glucose.

Note that some of these symptoms are also seen in epilepsy and this may lead to delay in diagnosis in a person with both conditions. This is because the recovery may appear to be because of the administration of glucose correcting the hypoglycaemia, and not spontaneous from seizure activity.

EPILEPSY TYPES AND CAUSES

Idiopathic

The only true idiopathic epilepsy is primary generalized. This is where no localized onset is seen on electroencephalograph, with changes seen on all channels during the seizure. There are no underlying causes.

Cryptogenic

This form of epilepsy will present as partial onset with or without secondary generalization. There is an underlying cause to this type of seizure, although it may not always be identifiable.

With the introduction of MRI scans, it is now possible to identify areas of cerebral damage that were previously undetectable. However, this does not always result in any change in treatment. Often the treatment of the seizures with anti-epileptic drugs is still the only appropriate therapy. The improved detection will, however, result in better prognostic indicators.

Symptomatic

This is where a definite underlying cause is found. This cause may or may not need to be treated. In some cases, the treatment of the underlying cause may result in a cessation of the seizure activity.

In children it may be linked to:

- Congenital abnormalities
- Birth trauma
- CNS infection
- Febrile convulsions.

At any age it may be linked to cerebral trauma – accidental or surgical.

In the elderly it may be linked to cerebrovascular disease – e.g. stroke, repeated TIA.

Intracranial tumours can be a cause of epilepsy. This is more common in adults than in children because of the different tumour types found at different ages.

> Although the classification of epilepsy appears complex, it is worth bearing in mind that there are only two types of epilepsy: focal in onset, and generalized. Either the seizure starts in a localized part of the brain, or the whole brain goes straight into a seizure (primary generalized). There are many epilepsy syndromes, but the diagnosis is complex and is made by specialists.

TYPES OF SEIZURES

Partial seizures

Simple

In partial seizures the consciousness is not impaired and the person is usually able to respond.

The altered cerebral activity will be very localized, and any symptoms experienced will depend on the area of the brain affected. These symptoms may be motor or sensory, e.g. tingling in one part of the body, various types of hallucinations, twitching of one limb or one side of the face.

These seizures are often referred to by the person as a 'warning' or 'aura'. They are not always recognized as seizures, but still preclude the person from legally holding a driving licence.

This type of seizure is usually short, lasting seconds to minutes, with rapid recovery.

This type of seizure can be mistaken for tics, mental illness, or transient ischaemic attack.

Complex partial

In complex partial seizures, although the person may appear alert, consciousness is impaired. The person is confused and unlikely to respond, or will respond inappropriately, and may carry out repetitive actions such as plucking at clothing, fiddling with objects nearby, or pulling the hair (automatisms). During the seizure the person may wander around, and if restrained may become aggressive or respond violently because he or she will not recognize familiar people or surroundings. Prior to these episodes the person may report a characteristic warning (aura). This may be a noise, strange smell or taste, or a feeling of *déjà vu*.

This type of seizure can last from a few minutes up to a few hours. Some patients may experience seizures occurring intermittently for a whole day.

This type of seizure may be mistaken for drunkenness, drug abuse, hypoglycaemia, or mental illness.

Secondary generalized

Secondary generalized seizures can occur following either simple or complex seizures, and is when the localized activity spreads to become generalized. They usually result in a tonic–clonic seizure, although muscular twitching is not always seen.

In some people the partial element is not recognized, and they are thought to have primary generalized seizures.

This type of seizure may be mistaken for a faint (with twitching), cardiac arrhythmia, stroke, or non-epileptic attack.

Generalized seizures

Tonic–clonic

The onset of tonic–clonic seizures is usually abrupt. The person may cry out prior to falling, and then become stiff. Jerking, usually affecting the whole body, follows the rigid phase. Breathing may be affected, and some cyanosis may occur. When the jerking subsides, the person will be slow to recover, may be confused and may want to sleep. Incontinence may or may not occur.

The tonic–clonic phase usually lasts 1–3 minutes, although total recovery may take 20 minutes or longer. Some people may take hours to recover completely.

This type of seizure may be mistaken for a faint (with twitching), cardiac arrhythmia, or non-epileptic attack.

Generalized absence seizures (petit mal)

Generalized absence seizures present in children, and although they may continue into adulthood they do not initially present in adults. A seizure is sudden in onset; the child will stare into space and not respond. In some children, repeated blinking and swallowing may be seen. Recovery is rapid, and the child will continue with his or her activity. This type of seizure usually lasts from 5–20 seconds.

These absence seizures should not be confused with the absence seizures that can present in adults with temporal or frontal lobe epilepsy, as the drug of choice for treatment of each is different.

This type of seizure may be mistaken for daydreaming (dreamy kid at the back of the class), lack of attention, or a learning disability.

Myoclonic seizures

In myoclonic seizures, there is sudden onset of jerking movement of the limbs with or without trunkal involvement. It most commonly involves the upper limbs, although in some people only one limb may seem to be involved. The person may appear to drop or throw objects, or to knock objects over. Although there is loss of consciousness in these attacks, this may be so short that the person concerned does not realize. However, in some people the jerking may be severe and they may fall.

This form of epilepsy most commonly presents in children or

adolescents, and prior to diagnosis the child may be described as clumsy. Most episodes occur on waking. It is usually a benign form of epilepsy that responds quickly to treatment. This type of seizure is usually of short duration, lasting only seconds, although the seizures may cluster, leading to prolonged episodes. Often the child will present because of a tonic–clonic seizure that was thought to be a first episode.

History taking is, in this instance, very important, as myoclonic jerks may not be mentioned unless prompted. In many cases if treatment is discontinued the seizures will recur, and control may not be regained easily. Careful consideration is therefore necessary when determining the time for which treatment is required. Some figures quote a 90 per cent risk of seizures returning if medication is stopped. Adapting the person's lifestyle to avoid potential triggers may alter this.

There is a variant of this type of epilepsy that is progressive and will result in uncontrolled myoclonic and generalized seizures. This is a rare, drug-resistant form of epilepsy that is not suitable for surgical treatment.

This type of seizure may be mistaken for clumsiness or other causes of lack of co-ordination.

Tonic and atonic seizures

In both tonic and atonic seizures, the seizures are sudden in onset and the person will fall abruptly to the floor. Loss of consciousness is very short and may not be recognized; recovery is often rapid, with the person wanting to continue his or her previous activity.

In tonic seizures, there is sudden stiffening of the trunk and the person will fall like a log. Injury to the head is therefore common.

In atonic seizures, there is sudden loss of muscle tone and the person will crumple to the floor. Injury may therefore be less common.

These seizures usually last only seconds, and recovery is rapid if injury has not occurred.

These types of seizure may be mistaken for a faint or cataplexy.

Photosensitive epilepsy

This is genetically related epilepsy, and is often triggered by sensitivity to specific frequencies of flickering lights. This type of epilepsy is often treated as an indication of the presence of primary generalized epilepsy; on EEG, changes may be seen on the occipital lobe before any generalized spread is seen.

Only approximately 25 per cent of children will be photosensitive.

Other trigger factors can be specific patterns (usually lines or grids), combinations of certain bright colours, word formations, or type patterns (reading epilepsy).

Having this form of epilepsy does not necessarily mean that a child cannot use a computer. By working in a well-lit room, altering contrasts between background and text, adjusting colour combinations, and avoiding rapidly moving games, a computer can still be used.

Careful consideration is necessary when determining the time for which treatment is required, because of the high risk of seizures recurring if treatment is withdrawn. Adapting the person's lifestyle to avoid potential triggers may alter this.

EPILEPSY SYNDROMES

An epilepsy syndrome is usually age related, and can be classified by:

- Age of onset
- A collection of symptoms
- Specific EEG characteristics.

Owing to the complexity of the epilepsy syndromes and the specialist knowledge needed in dealing with these, we will consider them only briefly in this book. Many syndromes will also be associated with some degree of learning disability, and will have been present from childhood. Many involve multiple seizure types and refractory epilepsy, even on polytherapy. In many cases the support will need to be multidisciplinary, as these syndromes may also include behavioural problems – such as the West syndrome (infantile spasms) and the Lennox–Gastaut syndrome.

Other epilepsy types may also be considered as syndromes and may not involve learning disability. Some may become progressive, and these include juvenile myoclonic epilepsy, benign myoclonic epilepsy and neonatal seizures.

INVESTIGATING EPISODES OF LOSS OF CONSCIOUSNESS

It is important to remember that the diagnosis of epilepsy is still, even in these days of advanced technology, mainly a clinical judgement. The history, lack of findings of other causes of loss of consciousness and altered perceptions are often the only indications that lead to the fact that this is the correct diagnosis.

Most investigations are performed to exclude any underlying pathology needing immediate treatment, or to establish co-morbidity that may or may not require treatment. The second criterion may be important in influencing prognosis outcomes or treatment pathways.

On many occasions investigations are carried out after the diagnosis is established, and not to aid in making the diagnosis. It is often this aspect that patients find difficult to understand, and the rationale for undertaking investigations is not always adequately explained.

Initial investigations

Initial investigations may include:

1. To check general medical condition in primary care:
   - physical examination
   - routine blood profile, including glucose
   - urine testing.
2. Specifically to establish epilepsy/seizure type in secondary care:
   - standard electroencephalogram (EEG)
   - sleep-deprived EEG
   - ambulatory EEG monitoring
   - videotelemetry
   - invasive electrodes.

Standard electroencephalogram

This is a short recording of the electrical activity of the brain using surface electrodes, usually lasting about 30 minutes (Figure 6.1).

If the person is having intermittent episodes, this recording may be normal. *A normal recording does not rule out epilepsy.*

Some EEGs may identify subtle changes in brainwave patterns; this is not always an indication of epilepsy. Occasionally an EEG will be frankly epiletogenic, but the patient may never have had and never will have a clinical seizure.

The EEG may be more useful in determining the type of epilepsy or a possible syndrome in a person with a definite diagnosis. This will in turn help to determine treatment plans and prognosis.

Sleep-deprived EEG

The aim of this test is to enable a recording to take place during normal sleep; it is not necessarily to estimate the effect of lack of sleep. It may be performed when the standard EEG has shown some non-specific changes.

The patient is deprived of sleep for a set number of hours, and then attends for the recording to be performed. A more prolonged recording will be undertaken as the patient becomes drowsy and then sleeps, and a further period of recording is then undertaken during sleep and continued as the patient is roused.

In this form of recording, slight changes may become more defined or their type become more identifiable.

Ambulatory EEG monitoring

This is undertaken when there is a definite diagnosis but control has not been established, or where there is some doubt about the number and type of attacks that the person is reporting in a set time span. It is particularly useful when a patient has both epilepsy and non-epileptic attacks and the dominant seizure type is not known. The patient is fitted with scalp electrodes, which are attached to a recording box. This is a portable system, and in most cases the patient does not have to stay in hospital. The diary kept during the recording is an essential part of this investigation.

Videotelemetry

In videotelemetry, the patient is videotaped and a continuous EEG is recorded at the same time. This is undertaken in hospital, and the idea is to capture an attack on video so the phenomenology of the attack can be compared with the EEG

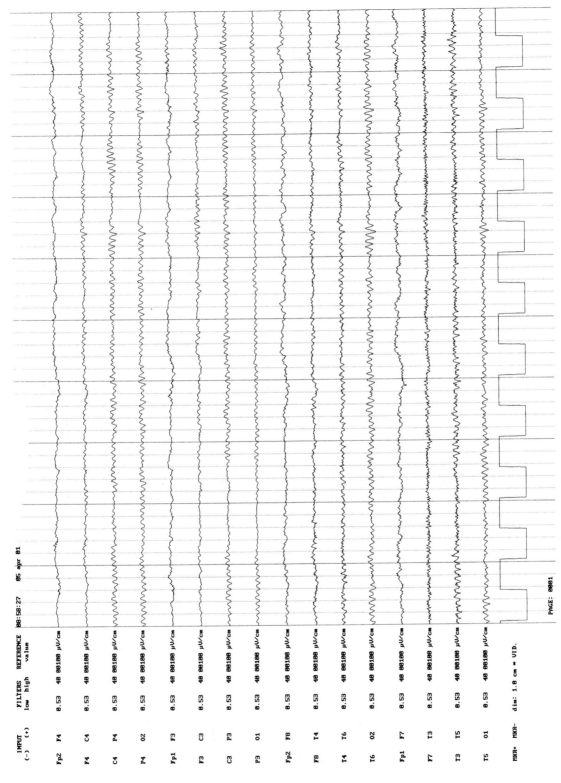

Figure 6.1 Normal EEG (electroencephalogram).

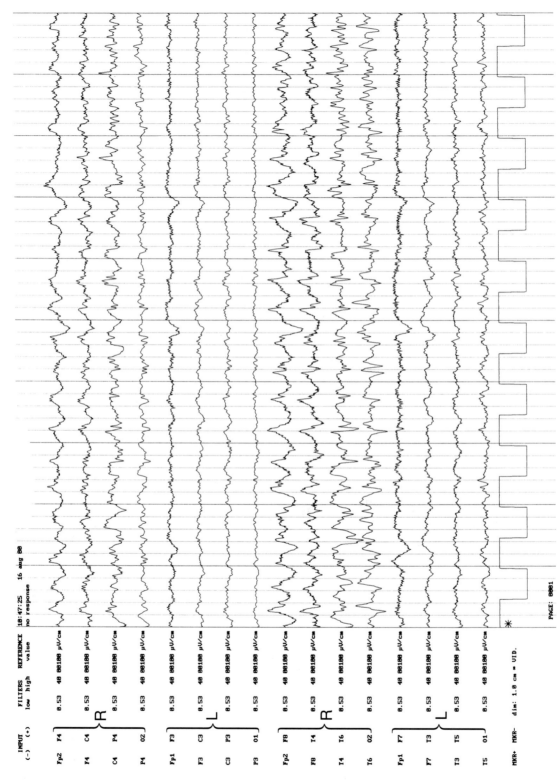

Figure 6.2 Focal onset seizure. Note: the right temporal leads (T4–T6, T6–O2) illustrate the greatest abnormality.

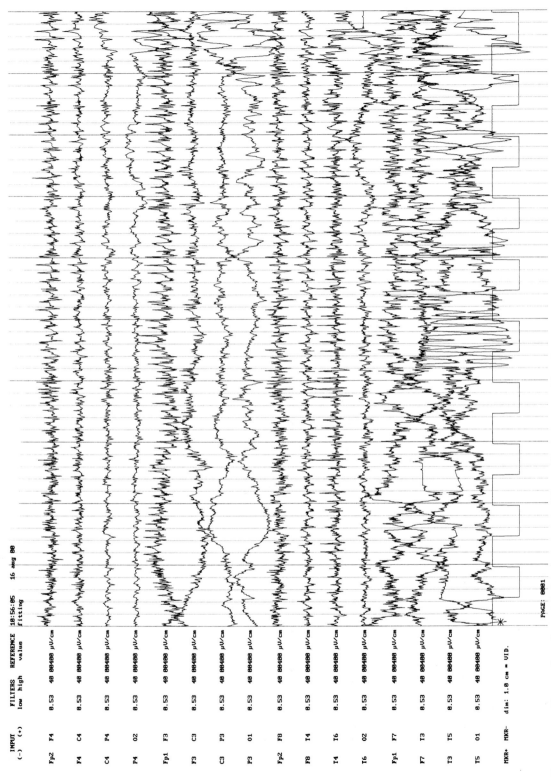

Figure 6.3 Generalized tonic–clonic seizure. Trace illustrates mid-seizure pattern.

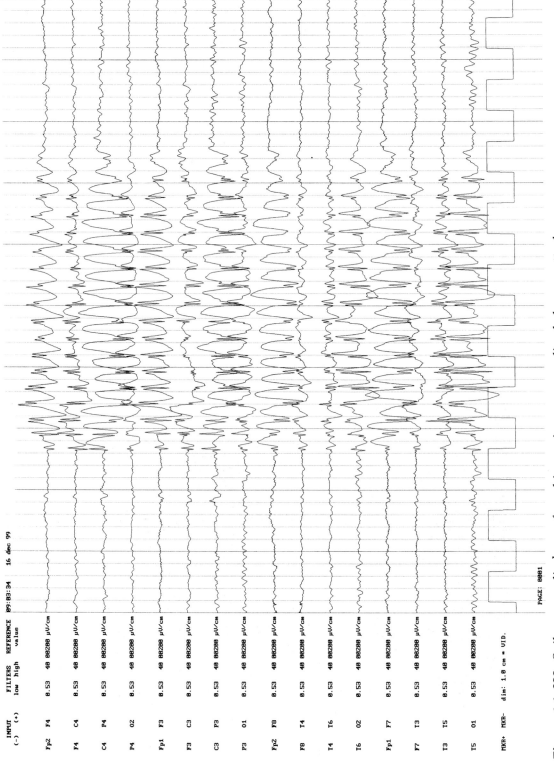

Figure 6.4 3Hz Spike-wave discharge found in a primary generalized absence attack.

findings. Sometimes patients will have their anti-epileptic drugs reduced so that it becomes more likely that an attack will occur and be captured on video. Videotelemetry is useful for evaluation of non-epilepsy attack syndrome, and also when patients are being evaluated for epilepsy surgery.

Invasive electrodes

Invasive electrodes are often used in conjunction with videotelemetry in specialist epilepsy centres, usually as part of the evaluation for epilepsy surgery. These can consist of sphenoidal electrodes, where electrodes are placed nearer to the temporal lobe than can be achieved with scalp electrodes, or the electrodes can be placed neurosurgically within the skull vault, on the surface of the brain.

Other investigations in secondary care

Neuroimaging

This is relevant in most people developing a seizure disorder, although it may be performed at different times in the diagnos-

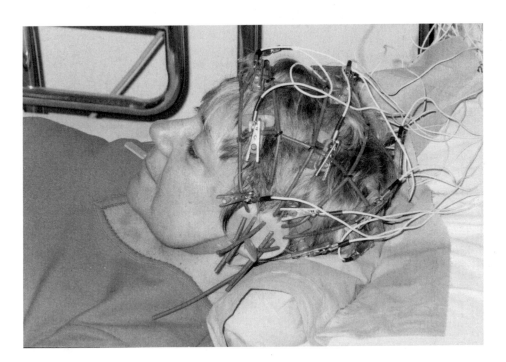

Figure 6.5 Photograph of person with EEG leads in place.

tic or monitoring stages of the condition depending on the age of the person, the presentation of the condition, and the type of seizure.

If there is evidence of some underlying structural lesion, acute illness or cerebral insult, then computed tomography (CT) scanning will probably be performed as soon as possible.

Seizure type may also influence the decision to perform a CT scan, as it may be of less benefit where the presentation is one of generalized tonic–clonic seizures than in partial seizures.

Some underlying structural causes of epilepsy may not be seen on CT scanning, although they may require surgical intervention. If possible, magnetic resonance imaging (MRI) is the investigation of choice for all patients with epilepsy, but cost and availability limit its use. In addition, MRI does not expose the patient to ionizing radiation, so it is preferable in children.

CT scanning

CT scanning is usually performed to eliminate any underlying structural lesion, e.g. a tumour or vascular problems. It is not

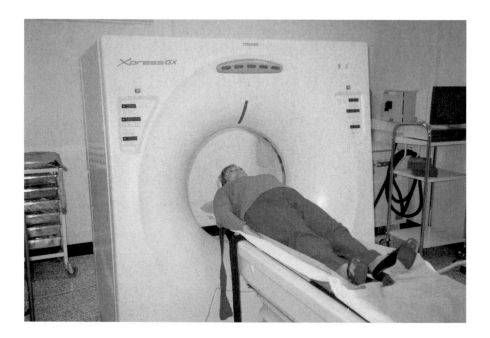

Figure 6.6 CT scanner. Undergoing this type of scan is less claustrophobic for the patient as the machine is open on both sides and only the subject's head enters the centre space. However, a CT scan is less informative than an MRI scan.

done to aid the diagnosis of epilepsy, and is of little use in helping to establish patients who may be suitable for surgical treatment of their seizures. For this reason, it may not be performed in patients with primary generalized epilepsy.

MRI scanning

MRI scanning can be used to establish focal lesions, which may be the trigger site for seizures. It is an essential part of establishing which patients are suitable for surgical treatment for their epilepsy. It should be performed on any patient presenting with temporal lobe epilepsy; especially where there is a history of repeated or prolonged febrile convulsions. It may also be useful in some patients with frontal lobe seizures. The decision regarding when to perform MRI scans will differ from patient to patient. The investigation is not always undertaken if the person becomes seizure-free on monotherapy or, in specific cases, on dual therapy. However, if control is not established, scanning should be performed within 2 years of onset of the seizures. Some people will need to be rescanned at intervals if the epilepsy remains uncontrolled.

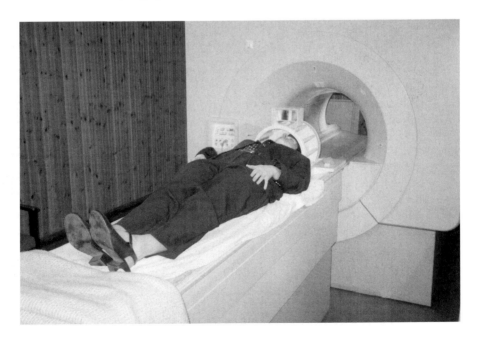

Figure 6.7 MRI scanner. With this type of scan the subject's whole body moves into the tunnel. Note the head coil in place: this improves the quality of the brain images.

THE IMPLICATIONS OF MAKING AN INCORRECT DIAGNOSIS

This is the most important aspect of providing the correct care in any condition, but in epilepsy the implications can be greater because of the complexities involved.

The seizures that present are merely a symptom, and not the condition itself. Added to this are other problems – is a seizure a seizure, or could it be a vaso-vagal attack or a cardiovascular event? When it is a seizure, is this idiopathic or symptomatic? If it is symptomatic, what treatment is needed?

Between 10 and 30 per cent of patients referred to specialist centres do not have epilepsy.

A correct diagnosis and classification will lead to correct treatment and help to predict long-term outcomes. This in turn will enable correct advice and support to be offered to the patient and carers, both professional and non-professional.

Incorrect diagnosis may lead either to the epilepsy not being correctly treated or to other conditions being left untreated. If it is not epilepsy, there are the additional implications of unnecessary medication being prescribed. There are also the social implications – the loss of a driving licence or employment, the effect on a child's education and in turn on their future prospects. Relationships may be affected in adults, and children may be denied the opportunity to learn social interactions.

The possibility of litigation

For the professional, making an incorrect diagnosis, providing incorrect advice, or not providing advice may all lead to litigation. You may not have been involved directly; it is important to remember that you are responsible for the actions of any person to whom you delegate a task. You should be sure that such a person is adequately trained, and has the appropriate knowledge to undertake the given task. People are responsible for their own actions if they do not inform you that they do not feel able to undertake the task, but you will ultimately be responsible. However, a mistake made in good faith is not negligence.

As nurses we are bound by the *Code of Professional Conduct* (UKCC, 1992a) and the *Scope of Professional Practice* (UKCC, 1992b), which state that we are responsible for our own actions and should not undertake tasks for which we are not trained. If we are to take on responsibilities previously within the remit of medical staff, then we need to ensure that we have adequate training. Having a little knowledge can be dangerous both for the patients and for us. Sometimes undertaking a specific English National Board (ENB) course does not provide sufficient training to take on certain roles. These courses may help to highlight areas in which we need to gain further education or act as a foundation for other training. We should not automatically be thought able to take on any task related to a condition because we have undertaken a course. We need to ensure that other staff understand this, seeking help and advice where necessary. Taking on activities for which we are not competent or adequately trained is negligent. Nurses taking on a role where the title includes the word 'specialist' must ensure that they have the experience not only academically but also clinically to deal with epilepsy.

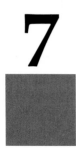

7

Special issues in diagnosis and treatment

NON-EPILEPTIC ATTACK DISORDER

The term 'non-epileptic attack disorder' (NEAD) is usually associated with seizures with a psychological cause, although it does also refer to any seizures that are not epileptogenic in nature and may have other medical causes, e.g. hypoglycaemia and vaso-vagal episodes.

Many cases are associated with severe psychological trauma – often abuse in childhood or adolescence. It may also be associated with unresolved bereavement. The different underlying causes may mean that various psychiatric and counselling services will need to be accessed for different patients – for example, rape crisis or bereavement counselling. Treatment may need to continue for years. Research seems to indicate that prognosis is better if contact with neurology services continues during the counselling.

The following points should be noted:

- In some situations it may be difficult to distinguish these seizures from epileptic seizures
- Seizures do not always occur at times of stress
- It is important to remember that in most situations the person having this type of seizure is not aware of the episode
- There is sometimes a misconception that the person is in control of his or her actions during a seizure
- The diagnosis of non-epileptic seizures is as difficult to make as the diagnosis of epilepsy
- This condition is often more difficult to treat than to diagnose
- If you are involved in trying to diagnose this condition, you will need to be aware of how treatment will be provided and how the patient and family will be supported

- This condition is more common in women than men
- It may commence in childhood or adolescence
- It may be associated with a history of childhood abuse, severe psychological trauma or acute episodes of stress, such as exams
- It may occur in patients who also have epilepsy
- Some temporal and frontal lobe seizures may be very difficult to distinguish from non-epileptic seizures.

Distinguishing psychological seizures from epileptogenic seizures

Psychological seizures may be more prolonged, lasting from minutes to hours, and they are often slower in onset. During such seizures:

- Partial awareness may be demonstrated, with resistance to eye opening
- Muscle tone may be flaccid
- The periods of motor activity may fluctuate in severity
- Semi-purposeful thrashing of all limbs may occur
- Prominent pelvic movements may occur
- Serum prolactin levels may be helpful if a blood sample can be taken during or immediately after a seizure (this is not useful during pregnancy because of naturally raised levels).

Recovery from psychological seizures is usually more rapid than from epileptogenic seizures.

Table 7.1 compares the presentation of epileptic and non-epileptic seizures.

Treatment

NEAD does not respond to anti-epileptic medication. It is treated with counselling and support, and sessions will need to be frequent initially. Contact with neurology services should be maintained if they were previously involved, as this will give some continuity of care. It is important that this continued contact does not give the wrong impression of a mistaken diagnosis, but helps to provide reassurance. Communication

Table 7.1 Comparing seizure presentation

	Epilepsy	Non-epileptic seizures
Age of onset	Any age	Less common in the elderly
Warning/aura	May occur	May occur
Trigger	May have specific trigger; usually present immediately prior to the seizure	Usually emotional, although not always present at the time of the seizure
Duration	Usually short; complex seizures may be prolonged	Usually prolonged; may last for hours
Seizure activity	Usually stereotyped May be partial or generalized Automatism may occur May remain conscious May be unresponsive May be confused Pupils may be dilated May be vocal Pelvic thrusting uncommon but may occur in frontal lobe seizures	Not always stereotyped Usually generalized, although may present as absence seizure Does not usually involve automatism May respond during seizure Eyes resistant to opening Pupil's react May be vocal Pelvic thrusting more common
Timing	Seizures occur at any time May be associated with sleep Some people can induce seizures for attention	Seizures usually occur when witnesses are present Less common during sleep
Patient awareness	May have post-ictal drowsiness or headache Will usually give consistent report of pre- and post-seizure experience	Description may vary Post-ictal symptoms are rare
Incontinence	May occur	May occur
Injury	May occur depending on where seizure occurs	May occur, but usually in unwitnessed seizures
Suggestibility to episode occurring	Very unusual	May be triggered following suggestion
EEG findings	May be normal if done inter-ictally Changes will usually be seen if done during seizure Frontal lobe or deep-seated focus may not be recordable with scalp electrode EEG	Will be normal if done inter-ictally Will be normal if done during seizure May be difficult to interpret; movement may mask background recording

between professionals will be vital to ensure that correct treatment is maintained if the person also has a diagnosis of epilepsy. Many patients will not become seizure-free despite diagnosis and counselling. Treatment is more likely to be successful if contact is maintained with neurological services while other treatment is undertaken. In addition, it is important for health care professionals to be aware of the possibility of epileptic attacks also being present.

Dealing with non-epileptic seizures

- Deal with as for any other seizure
- Do not make a fuss
- Some non-epileptic seizures may present as generalized seizures; some may present as a partial seizure with the person able to talk during the episode but no automatism seen
- Ensure that the person is not in any danger
- If appropriate, place in the recovery position
- Talk to and reassure the person during the seizure, even if they seem unresponsive
- Let the person recover in his or her own time
- Do not make the person feel that he or she is being a nuisance
- Provide counselling and support
- Treatment with anti-epileptic medication is not appropriate
- Treat the patient with respect and courtesy.

Problems of misdiagnosis

Misdiagnosis may lead to:

- Inappropriate treatment with anti-epileptic medication
- The risk of inappropriate admission to intensive care with anaesthesia and ventilation, which can in itself involve life-threatening procedures
- Lack of appropriate treatment and access to counselling and psychological support.

STATUS EPILEPTICUS

Many medical and nursing staff may only be aware of the condition of convulsive status epilepticus. There are, however, many other forms of this condition, including:

- Absence status
- Non-convulsive simple partial status
- Complex partial status
- Myoclonic status in coma
- Myoclonic status in other forms of epilepsy
- Status epilepticus in mental retardation.

In this section we will discuss issues associated with tonic–clonic status. This is a life-threatening condition and is a true medical emergency. The treatment is usually shared management between anaesthetic and neurology services. Nursing input into the care of these patients will be either in an emergency setting or in an intensive care unit monitoring the person's progress. Where correct and speedy treatment is not available, the outcome can be poor.

As treatment for epilepsy has improved, the incidence of status epilepticus may be more common in people with no previous history of seizures than in those with an established diagnosis.

Possible underlying causes include:

- Cerebral trauma
- Cerebral tumour
- Cerebrovascular disease
- Intercranial infection (e.g. meningitis or encephalitis)
- Acute metabolic disturbance.

Medical complications of status epilepticus

Table 7.2 shows the medical complications of status epilepticus.

The treatment of status epilepticus

This model (Table 7.3) is taken from one developed by Professor Simon Shorvon of the Institute of Neurology, National Hospital for Nervous Diseases, London.

Table 7.2 Medical complications of status epilepticus

Cerebral	Cardiorespiratory	Metabolic	Other
Hypoxia	Hypotention	Dehydration	Multi-organ failure
Seizure-induced damage	Hypertension	Electrolyte disturbance; hyponatraemia/ hyperkalaemia/ hypoglycaemia	Fractures
Oedema	Cardiac failure	Acute renal failure	Infection
Raised intercranial pressure	Respiratory failure	Acute hepatic failure	Thrombophlebitis
Cerebral venous thrombosis	Pulmonary oedema	Acute pancreatitis	
Cerebral haemorrhage/ infarction	Hypopyrexia		
	Peripheral ischaemic		

Reasons for failure of emergency drug treatment to control seizures in generalized status epilepticus

- Inadequate emergency anti-epileptic drug therapy (administration of drugs at too low a dose)
- Failure to initiate maintenance anti-epileptic drug therapy (seizures will recur as the effect of emergency drug therapy wears off)
- The presence of hypoxia, hypotension, cardio-respiratory failure, metabolic disturbances
- Failure to identify medical complications (hyperthermia, hepatic failure, renal failure)
- Misdiagnosis (psychologically determined 'seizure', pseudostatus, may be almost as common as status epilepticus in specialist practice.

COMPLEX PARTIAL STATUS

Diagnosis and treatment of complex partial status

Nursing input into the treatment of this type of status may differ from that in tonic–clonic status. Patients may not be admitted to

Table 7.3 Treatment of status epilepticus

0–10 minutes	0–60 minutes	60–90 minutes	>90 minutes
Assess cardio-respiratory function	Start emergency anti-epileptic medication	Establish aetiology	If seizures continue, patient must be transferred to intensive care unit
Secure airway	Start regular monitoring	Establish previous history of epilepsy	Establish intensive care monitoring
Resuscitate where necessary	Neurological observation	If AEDs have been withdrawn, reintroduce as rapidly as possible	Initiate EEG monitoring to assess cerebral activity compared to motor activity
Administer oxygen	Blood pressure, pulse, temperature, ECG	No previous history: investigate and treat underlying cause	EEG monitoring should be undertaken on a daily basis until no epileptogenic activity is seen
	Set up intravenous lines for fluid replacement and drug administration. IV access should be through large veins	Initiate emergency drug treatment	If status is not controlled within 90 minutes, full anaesthesia is required. Attempts to control seizures in sub-anaesthetic doses are unlikely to be effective
	Drugs should not be mixed; separate lines are needed for each drug	Identify and treat medical complications	Further delay may result in cerebral damage
	Take bloods for biochemical gases, pH, clotting, haematology, toxicology, virology	Give pressure therapy where appropriate	Full ITU and EEG facilities are required during anaesthesia
	Administer glucose (50 ml of 50% solution) and/or intravenous thiamine where appropriate	Initiate long-term maintenance drug therapy in tandem with emergency treatment. Choice of drug will depend on type of epilepsy	

hospital for treatment, and the nurse can act as a contact to help in monitoring the progress of the treatment. The nurse can also liaise between the specialist, the patient and the GP to ensure that recommended changes of medication are acted upon.

Complex partial status occurs when there is a prolonged epileptic episode in which fluctuating or frequently recurring epileptic cerebral discharges result in a confused state. It is not usually in itself life threatening.

- It is most likely to occur in patients with temporal or frontal lobe epilepsy, but can present in any type of partial epilepsy
- It usually lasts for several hours, but may last for days or weeks
- Episodes of this type of status are often recurrent in the patient and may occur periodically
- The presentation will depend on the site of the epileptic focus
- There may be confusion and this may fluctuate
- It may be difficult in some patients to distinguish the symptoms of partial status from some symptoms of drug toxicity
- EEG monitoring is needed to diagnose these conditions
- A cause may not be identified, but it may be due to infection or sudden drug changes
- Oral treatment with barbiturates may be used initially; it may be necessary to administer intravenous barbiturates if the seizures continue or the patient becomes distressed
- EEG monitoring will be necessary to evaluate progress in order to assess when barbiturate treatment can be withdrawn
- Permanent neurological deficit is rare.

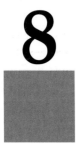

8

Epilepsy treatment

INTRODUCTION

In this chapter we will discuss some of the main aspects of treatment for epilepsy. This will include basic information on some drugs used. For more details on all the drugs available you should consult individual data sheets or the *British National Formulary* (BNF, 2001), though this does not always contain all the information available. Also included in the chapter is information on other forms of treatment.

The use of anti-epileptic drugs

Prescribing issues in the treatment of epilepsy

Using drugs in specialist units

In specialist units, drugs may be used outside the recommendations of the drug company or the *BNF*. This can result in a prescribing issue, as some GPs may be reluctant to issue prescriptions for drugs that they are not familiar with or at doses that are higher than those recommended in the licence issued for the drug.

Brand *v.* generic prescribing

Most drugs have at least two names, a branded name and a generic name (e.g. brand, Valium; generic, diazepam). Owing to the increasing cost of health care, generic prescribing has now become standard practice in both primary and secondary care. Hospital doctors write prescriptions using the generic name, and the pharmacy will usually choose the cheapest preparation for the patient. Many computers used to issue repeat prescriptions in primary care will automatically transpose drugs to their generic name when entered.

There is evidence that brand changing in the use of AEDs can result in loss of seizure control or the onset of side effects. The results of the research are questioned by some, but in clinical practice there is much anecdotal evidence to support it. The bioavailability (the amount of the drug that gets into the system) may vary between two brands by up to 20 per cent. Because of the narrow therapeutic window of AEDs, any change of brand can potentially result in problems. An additional factor is the large number of generic brands of some drugs, which could result in multiple changes occurring.

Patients can be confused by the information given, as specialist nurses will usually advise them about these potential problems although pharmacists will often tell them that they are being given the same drug and it is not a problem.

In the *British National Formulary*, some drugs now do have comments added referring to varying bioavailability and pharmacokinetics. Advice is given that it may be prudent to avoid changing the formulation prescribed – e.g. carbamazepine and phenytoin.

When to start treatment

Before any drug therapy is commenced, it is very important to ensure that the correct diagnosis has been reached.

Treatment is not usually started following an isolated seizure. There may, however, be some exceptions to this. For example, if a person presents with a first generalized tonic–clonic seizure but the history is suggestive of partial seizures or myoclonus in the past, then treatment is started following this first tonic–clonic seizure.

Which drugs to use

The correct classification of epilepsy and seizure types will play an important part in choosing the correct medication, as some forms of epilepsy may be aggravated by some AEDs (e.g. carbamazepine in primary generalized seizures).

The age and sex of the patient are also influencing factors if more than one drug is suitable. The drug of choice may differ when dealing with a young female patient from the one chosen for a young male patient or for an elderly patient, although they may all have the same epilepsy and seizure type. For example, it is usually recommended to avoid sodium valproate in young female patients because of the large number of side effects, its potential impact on fertility, and foetal abnormalities.

First-line drugs

First-line drugs are usually licensed for use as monotherapy. Most of these drugs are well established and have been licensed for many years. However, it is now recognized that some of them have unacceptable side effects when taken long term. They are still used, but only in specific situations or when other therapy has failed (e.g. phenytoin for status epilepticus or chronic refractory epilepsy).

When commencing treatment, a single drug should be prescribed, starting with a low dose and gradually increasing this until the seizures are controlled or side effects present. If side effects present before control is achieved or the seizures are not controlled on the maximum dose tolerated by the patient or that recommended in the *British National Formulary*, then an alternative drug will need to be tried. This will usually be another first-line drug. If all suitable first-line drugs fail, then a second-line drug will need to be added. In each of these situations the chosen drug should be added at a low dose and increased slowly. If the seizures were controlled on two first-line drugs but as one is withdrawn the seizures recur, then the first drug should be reintroduced. This process may need to be repeated with more than one first-line drug.

Second-line drugs

Second-line drugs are those licensed for use in conjunction with a monotherapy drug. In clinical practice you may have contact with people only on second-line drugs. This is not uncommon if the person is under the care of a specialist; it can occur if seizure control is achieved and the first-line drug can be withdrawn.

If seizure control has not been achieved with a single drug or a combination of first-line drugs, then a second-line drug should be introduced in combination with the most effective first-line drug. Again the drug should be gradually increased up to the recommended or maximum tolerated dose. If this regimen fails to obtain seizure control, this drug should be reduced and discontinued and another second-line drug tried.

Drug dosing regimens

Although all manufacturers recommend a start, maintenance and maximum dose for their drug, these are only guidelines. All regimens should be tailored to the individual. In clinical practice specialists will sometimes use drugs outside the manufacturer's guidelines in accordance with their own clinical experience. It should be remembered that the correct dose for any patient is one that controls the seizures without producing unwanted side effects. This may be a low dose, or one at the top of the dose range.

On some occasions seizure control is not possible without incurring unwanted side effects. If this is the case, the patient should be given the choice. Some will prefer to have no seizures even with drug side effects, whereas others will want to eliminate unwanted side effects at the risk of continuing to have seizures.

We should be providing the information to enable patients to make their own choice.

Which drugs for which seizures

Tables 8.1 and 8.2 provide basic information on some of the commonly used and newer first- and second-line anti-epileptic medications. Tables 8.3 and 8.4 give further details regarding their half-life, time to peak levels and some significant interactions. Fuller information on all AEDs follows. For further information on drugs and their interactions, please refer to the *BNF* or individual drug data sheets.

Individual drug information

The starting and incremental dosing in the following information includes the regimen used within our unit where the

Table 8.1 Drugs licensed as first-line treatment

Drug	Normal role	Avoid in	Comment
Carbamazepine Tegretol Tegretol Retard Teril CR Timonil Retard	Adults and children All types of partial seizures Secondary generalized seizures	Myoclonic epilepsy Generalized absence seizures Patients with hepatic problems	Interaction with many drugs including other AEDs and NONE AEDs Oral contraception needs at least 50mcg oestrogen per day still not always effective Increased teretagenesis Folic acid 5 mg daily advised prior to pregnancy Advice Vitamin K 20 mg daily from 36/40 gestation May lower thyroxin levels Monitor for onset of skin rash Increased incidence of impotence
*Lamotrigine Lamictal	Adults and children Partial seizures and generalization Primary generalized seizures Myoclonus	Hepatic, renal and clotting parameters should be monitored	Interacts with sodium valproate, carbamazepine and other enzyme inducing drugs
Phenytoin Epanutin	Adults and children As for carbamazepine Status epilepticus	Most circumstances Absence seizures Women of child bearing age Young patients	Now more usually used as emergency treatment for uncontrolled seizures or when all other drugs have failed Interacts with oral contraceptive Often well tolerated
Sodium Valproate Epilim Convulex	Adults and children Generalized seizures including myoclonus and generalized absence seizures	Young females Women of child bearing age	Interacts with many AED's and other drugs Increased teretagenesis Weight gain Hair loss
Ethosuxamide Zarontin Emeside	Children Generalized absence seizures	Children with gastric problems	Now not so commonly used, Sodium Valproate replacing this drug

*Lamotrigine is now licensed as a first-line drug, but is often only used when a more traditional first-line drug has been tried.

Table 8.2 Drugs licensed as second-line treatment

Drug	Mormal role	Avoid in	Comment
Gabapentin Neurontin	In adults All types of partial seizures Secondary generalized seizures	None known	Relatively new drug, all problems not yet known No apparent interactions May exacerbate seizures in some people Initially was used at too low a dose with limited efficacy
Levetiracetam Kepra	In adults All partial seizures with or without secondary generalist	Recently licensed only limited experience in clinical practice	No interactions reported May be useful in myoclonic and primary seizures Drowsiness often passes after a couple of weeks
Oxcarbazepine Trileptal (Also licensed for monotherapy use)	In adults All partial with or without secondary seizures	Impaired renal function	Interaction with oral contraceptive Treat as carbamazepine when using
Tiagabine Gabitril	In adults All partial seizures Secondary generalized seizures	Previous history of psychiatric or behavioural problems	One of the newer AEDs; limited experience Seems to be associated with increased headache
Topiramate Topamax	Adults and children All types of partial seizures Generalized tonic clonic seizures Lennox–Gastaut syndrome	Previous history of behavioural or psychiatric problems	Increased risk of renal stones May cause gastric upset Weight loss Interacts with oral contraceptive
Vigabatrin Sabril	All types of partial seizures Infantile spasms Lennox–Gastaut	Previous history of behavioural problems	Causes irreversible peripheral visual field loss

Table 8.3 The elimination half-life and time to peak levels of AEDs

Drug	Time to peak levels	Elimination half-life
Carbamazepine	4–8 hours	5–26 hours
Clobazam	1–4 hours	10–50 hours
Clobazepam	1–4 hours	20–80 hours
Ethosuximide	< 4 hours	30–69 hours
Felbamate	1–4 hours	20 hours(13–30 hours*)
Gabapentin	2–4 hours	5–9 hours
Lamotrigine	1–3 hours	30 hours (15 hours* 60 hours**)
Levetiracetam	0.6–1.3 hours	6–8 hours
Oxcarbazepine	4–5 hours	8–10 hours
Phenobarbitone	1–3 hours(variable)	75–120 hours
Phenytoin	4–12 hours	7–42 hours(mean 20 hours depending on serum levels)
Piracitam	30–40 minutes	5–6 hours
Primidone	3 hours	5–18 hours (75–120 hours derived phenobarbitone)
Tiagabine	1 hour	3.8–4.9 hours
Topiramate	2 hours	18–23 hours(varies depending on combined therapy)
Valproate	1–8 hours(depends on formulation)	4–12 hours
Vigabatrin	2 hours	4–7 hours

*Half-life when added to enzyme-inducing drugs
**Half-life when added to valproate.

recommendations within the *BNF* have been found to be inappropriate for many people. For manufacturers guidelines, see *BNF*.

Carbamazepine

Brand names: Tegretol, Tegretol Retard, Tetril CR, Timonil Retard.
Licensed in 1965, used for adults and children, for all forms of seizures except generalized absence. It is not recommended for the treatment of myoclonic epilepsy, as it does appear to have an adverse effect on this type of seizure. It is also used as pain control for neuropathy pain.
Usual preparations:

Tablets	100, 200, 400 mg
Chewtabs	100, 200 mg

Table 8.4 Significant interactions of AEDs

Drug	Significant interactions
Carbamazepine	Lamotrigine, oral contraceptives, thyroxine
Clobazam	Minor interactions common, not usually clinically significant
Clonazepame	Minor interactions common, not usually clinically significant
Ethosuximide	Levels increased by valproate, reduced by carbamazepine, phenytoin and phenobarbital
Felbamate	Increases levels of carbamazepine epoxide, phenytoin, phenobarbital and valproate
	Lowers concentration of carbamazepine, phenytoin, phenobarbital
	Carbamazepines lowers felbamate levels
	Valproates increases felbamate levels
Gabapentin	None
Lamotrigine	Phenytoin, carbamazepine
	Phenobarbital lowers lamotrigine levels
	Sodium valproate increases lamotrigine levels
	Lamotrigine increases metabolite retention of carbamazepine
Levetiracetam	None
Oxcarbazepine	Fewer than carbamazepine
Phenobarbital	Interacts with many drugs (AEDs and others)
Phenytoin	Interacts with many drugs (AEDs and others)
Piracetam	None
Primidone	Many in common with phenobarbital
Tiagabine	Levels lowered by carbamazepine, phenytoin, phenobarbital
Topiramate	Levels lowered by carbamazepine, phenytoin, phenobarbital
Valproate	Interacts with many drugs (AEDs and others)
Vigabatrin	Lowers phenytoin levels

Slow-release	200, 400 mg
Liquid	100 mg in 5 ml
Suppositories	125, 250 mg

Dose regimen:

Recommended starting dose in adults	100 mg daily
Incremental doses (our local use)	100 mg every 2 weeks until seizures stop or a maximum tolerated dose is reached
Maintenance doses	600–2000 mg daily

Maximum adult dose   2400 mg daily
Decremental doses   As for incremental
                                   doses in reverse

Most common maintenance dose:
Adults   400–1600 mg per day.
Children <1 year   100–200 mg daily
Children 1–5 years   200–400 mg daily
Children 5–10 years   400–600 mg daily
Children 10–15 years   600–1000 mg daily
Usual dose intervals:
Adults   Two to three divided doses per day
Children   Two to four divided doses per day
Serum level monitoring: Useful if used in conjunction with clinical information.
Target range: This may vary depending on the laboratory used. You need know your lab's normal values, often 4–12 mg/ml or 20–50 µmol/l.
Side effects: Drowsiness, sedation, dizziness, fatigue, ataxia, skin rash, visual disturbance, headache, insomnia, gastro-intestinal disturbance, impotence, mood swings, behavioural disturbance, hepatic disturbance, bone marrow dyscrasias, hyponatraemia, fluid retention, nephritis, Stevens–Johnson syndrome.
Method of excretion: Hepatic.
Contraindications: Patients with atrioventricular abnormalities; patients on monoamine-oxidase inhibitors or within 2 weeks of monoamine-oxidase inhibitor therapy.
Important interactions: Hormonal contraceptives. Patients on these should be taking a preparation containing at least 50 µg of oestrogen to obtain adequate levels for contraception, and may need to either take more than this or tri-cycle the packs (see current *BNF* for reference).
Warfarin and thyroxin levels may be lowered.
Reported teratogenic effects: Neural tube defect, cardiac defects, cleft palate.
Note: Tegretol Retard is a modified-release form of carbamazepine. The same guidelines should be followed as for carbamazepine. In some patients, higher doses can be achieved on this preparation without unwanted side effects.

Ethosuximide

Brand names: Zarontin, Emeside.
Licensed in 1958 for use in primary generalized absence

seizures (petit mal), which are usually seen in children and do not present in adults.

Usual preparation:

Capsules	250 mg
Syrup	250 mg/5 ml

Dose regimen:

Recommended starting dose in adults	250 g daily
Recommended starting dose in children	10–15 mg/kg per day

Maintenance dose:

Adults	750–2000 mg per day
Children	20–40 mg/kg per day
Decremental doses	As for incremental doses in reverse

Usual dose interval: Two to three divided doses per day.

Serum level monitoring: Useful if used in conjunction with clinical information.

Target range: Check for local laboratory normal values (40–100 mg/ml).

Side effects: Gastro-intestinal disturbance, weight loss, drowsiness, ataxia, headache, hiccups, depression, behavioural disturbance, acute psychotic reaction, rash, tremor, blood dyscrasia, systemic lupus erythematosus.

Method of excretion: Hepatic.

Important interactions: Ethosuximide levels raised by sodium valproate. Levels lowered by carbamazepine, phenytoin and phenobarbitol.

Gabapentin

Brand name: Neurontin.

Licensed in 1993 as add-on therapy for adults in the treatment of partial seizures with or without secondary generalization. It is not recommended for children. It is also used as pain control for neuropathic pain.

Usual preparation:

Capsules	100, 300, 400 mg
Tablets	600 mg, 800 mg

Dose regimen:

Recommended starting dose	300 mg
Incremental doses (our local use)	300 mg per week
Maintenance dose	900–3600 mg per day
Maximum dose	3600 mg per day
Decremental doses	As for incremental doses in reverse

Usual dose interval: Two to three divided doses per day.

Serum level monitoring: Not useful.

Side effects: Somnolence, dizziness, ataxia, fatigue, nystagmus, headache, tremor, nausea, vomiting, tremor, rhinitis, exacerbation of seizures.

Method of excretion: Renal.

Important interactions: None known.

Teratogenic effects: Because this is a relatively new drug there is little information available. It should be used with caution during pregnancy.

Note: When used in elderly patients or patients with renal impairment, it may be necessary to use reduced doses.

Lamotrigine

Brand name: Lamictal.

Licensed in 1991 for adults. Used as add-on therapy or monotherapy for partial and primary generalized seizures. Also licensed for children over 2 years for use as:

- Monotherapy in the treatment of partial, primary and secondary generalized tonic–clonic seizures
- Add-on therapy in the treatment of partial, primary and secondary generalized tonic–clonic seizures
- Add-on therapy for the treatment of partial, primary and secondary generalized seizures, and for seizures associated with Lennox–Gastaut syndrome, up to the age of 12 years.

Usual preparations:

Tablets	25, 50, 100, 200 mg
Chewtabs	5, 25, 100 mg

Dose regimen:

Recommended starting dose	12.5–25 mg daily
Incremental doses for adults (our local use)	25 mg every 2 weeks
Incremental doses for children	0.3 mg/kg every 2 weeks
Maintenance dose in adults	100–200 mg daily as monotherapy or with sodium valproate 200–400 mg daily in conjunction with carbamazepine, phenytoin

Maximum dose in adults(our local use)	400–800 mg daily
Maximum dose in children	5–15 mg/kg
Decremental doses	As for incremental doses in reverse

Usual dose intervals: In adults and children, two divided doses per day.

Serum level monitoring: Not often used as values are not definitely established. May be used in specific situations, e.g. pregnancy, if the patient's levels have been established during the seizure-free state.

Main side effects: Rash, headache, somnolence, dizziness, ataxia, fatigue, double vision, nausea, vomiting, tremor, psychosis, hypersensitivity reactions, blood dyscrasia.

Patients developing a rash, flu-like illness, fever, or worsening of seizures should have hepatic and renal function plus clotting factors monitored, as this could indicate Stevens–Johnson syndrome.

Method of excretion: Hepatic.

Contraindications: Patients with a history of hepatic impairment.

Important interactions: Lamotrigine interacts with sodium valproate, and dosing should be half that used in patients not on sodium valproate.

Lamotrigine has been found to cause retention of the metabolites of carbamizepine in some patients, and this can increase the risk of symptoms of toxicity. Drug level monitoring is not appropriate in this situation, as serum carbamizepine levels will often remain stable.

To counteract the symptoms, carbamizepine should be reduced by 100-mg increments until the symptoms abate, while closely monitoring seizure control.

Teratogenic effects: Because this is a relatively new drug as monotherapy, there is little information available.

Levetiracetam

Brand name: Kepra.

This new anti-epileptic drug was launched in the UK in November 2000, and is licensed for use as add-on therapy in partial epilepsy with or without secondary generalization. It may have potential for treating primary generalized seizures.

Usual preparation:

| Tablets | 250, 500, 750, 1000 mg |

Dose regimen:

Recommended starting dose	1000 mg daily
Incremental doses	500 mg every 2–4 weeks
Maintenance dose	1000–3000 mg daily
Maximum dose	3000 mg daily
Decremental doses	As for incremental doses in reverse

Some people may find this regimen inappropriate if they are already on polytherapy; 250 mg increments may be useful.

Usual dose interval: Two divided doses per day.

Serum level monitoring: Not relevant; values not established.

Main side effects: Somnolence, asthenia, infection, dizziness, headache.

Method of excretion: Partially hydrolysed in the blood to an inactive compound. Predominantly excreted unchanged from the kidneys.

Contraindications: None reported.

Important interactions: None reported.

Teratogenic effects: Insufficient use to be known.

Oxcarbazepine

Brand name: Trileptol.

This is a new anti-epileptic drug recently launched in the UK. It is licensed for use as add-on and monotherapy in partial epilepsy with or without secondary generalization. This drug has a similar mode of action to carbamizepine, but there is evidence that it is better tolerated.

Usual preparation:

Tablets	150, 300, 600 mg

Dose regimen:

Recommended starting dose	600 mg daily
Incremental doses	600 mg per week
Maintenance dose	900–2400 mg daily
Maximum dose	2400 mg daily
Decremental doses	As for incremental doses in reverse

Where this drug is being added to carbamazepine, the dose of carbamazepine may need to be reduced to avoid side effects. This can be done by substituting 150 mg of oxcarbazepine for 100 mg of carbamazepine.

Usual dose interval: Two divided doses per day.

Serum level monitoring: May be useful if used in conjunction with clinical information; values not established.

Target range: Check with local laboratory.

Main side effects: Main side effects as for carbamazepine, although oxcarbazepine is reported to be better tolerated. There is a higher incidence of hyponatraemia than seen in carbamazepine.

Method of excretion: Hydroxylation then conjugation.

Contraindications: As for carbamazepine.

Important interactions: Similar to carbamazepine, can cause problems of raised serum levels when added to carbamazepine.

Teratogenic effects: Not known due to insufficient clinical use, although probably similar to carbamazepine.

Phenobarbitol

Brand name: Phenobarbitone.

Licensed in 1912 as add-on and monotherapy for adults and children for all seizure types.

Usual preparation:

Tablets	15, 30, 50, 60, 100 mg
Elixir	15 mg/5 ml
Injection	200 mg/ml

Dose regimen:

Recommended starting dose for adults	30 mg per day
Recommended starting dose for children	3–6 mg/kg per day
Recommended starting dose for neonates	3–4 mg/kg per day
Incremental doses for adults	Increase gradually according to response
Maintenance for adults	30–180 mg daily
Decremental dose	Needs to withdrawn very slowly, depending on the length of time the person has been on the drug. Reductions may only be possible at 3-monthly intervals

Usual dose interval: One to two doses per day, usually at night if given once daily.

Serum level monitoring: Not often used; is measured as pheno-barbitone.

Target range: Check local normal values (e.g. 40–70 μmol/l phe-nobarbitone).

Main side effects: Acute dizziness, mood changes, aggression, cognitive dysfunction, dizziness, nausea, sedation, insomnia, hyperkinesis, impotence, reduced libido, folate deficiency, vita-mins K and D deficiency, osteomalacia, rash, connective tissue abnormality, frozen shoulder.

Method of excretion: Hepatic.

Important interactions: Most anti-epileptic medication, oral con-traceptives.

Teratogenic effects: Uncertain because of declining use, although advised to avoid use during pregnancy.

Note: Care needed when using in elderly people, or in children with impaired renal, hepatic or respiratory function. To be avoided during pregnancy. Breast-feeding is not advised if the mother is taking phenobarbitol.

Phenytoin

Brand names: Epanutin, Dilantin

Licensed in 1938 for all forms of seizures except absence. Due to the long-term side effect profile of this drug, it is now not com-monly used as one of the first choices of first-line therapy. It does however still have a place in the treatment of status, as it can be administered intravenously and the serum levels moni-tored to check effectiveness.

It is still also used in specific situations where daily dosing is beneficial – e.g. patients with memory problems or poor com-pliance. It is also licensed for children.

Usual preparation:

Capsules	25, 50, 100, 200 mg
Chewtabs	50 mg
Liquid suspension	30 mg/5 ml, 125 mg/5 ml
Injection	250 mg/5 ml

Dose regimen:

Recommended starting dose in adults	100–200 mg daily
Recommended starting dose in children	5 mg/kg
Incremental dose (our local use)	25–100 mg every 2–4 weeks until seizures stop or a maximum

	tolerated dose is reached
Maximum adult dose	300 mg daily, although higher doses may be tolerated by individuals
Decremental doses	Depends on the length of time that the person has been using the drug. There is a high risk of rebound seizures if withdrawn too quickly. Often reductions of 25 mg per month are used.

Most common maintenance dose:
Maintenance dose in adults   100–300 mg daily
Maintenance dose in children   4–8 mg/kg
Usual dose intervals: In adults and in children, one to two divided doses per day.
Serum level monitoring: Useful if used in conjunction with clinical information.
Target range: This may vary depending on the laboratory used. You need know your lab's normal values (often 10–20 mg/ml).
Main side effects: Ataxia, dizziness, lethergy, sedation, headache, dyskinesia, acute encephalopathy, hypersensitivity, rash, fever, blood dyscrasia, gum hyperplasia, folate deficiency, megablastic anaemia, vitamin K deficiency, thyroid dysfunction, decreased immunoglobins, mood changes, depression, coarsened facial features, hirsuteness, peripheral neuropathy, osteomalacia, hypocalcaemia, hormonal dysfunction, loss of libido, connective tissue alterations, hepititis, vasculitis, myopathy, coagulation defects, bone marrow hypoplasia.
Method of excretion: Hepatic.
Important interactions: Hormonal contraceptive – use as directed for patients on carbamazepine.
Sodium valproate – if these two drugs are used in combination, the CSF level of phenytoin can be raised without the serum level being affected. This will lead to toxic symptoms even when blood monitoring is showing satisfactory levels.

Teratogenic effects. Hare lip, foetal phenytoin syndrome.

Note: This is a very effective drug in the treatment of seizures, but can be very difficult to use as dose requirements will vary greatly between individuals. Because of the individual variations in the elimination of this drug and saturable metabolism, tolerance may vary in one individual at different times. What has been a stable and adequate dose may suddenly cause toxicity or loss of seizure control.

Patients can be so sensitive to changes in dosing that an alteration of 100 mg may induce a change from inadequate serum levels to toxicity. Changes of 25 mg per month may be all that some patients can tolerate.

Use is limited because of the number of short- and long-term side effects.

Piracetam

Brand name: Nootropil.

Used as add-on therapy to other AEDs for the treatment of myoclonus. Not recommended in children under 16 years of age.

Usual preparations:

Tablets	800, 1200 mg
Sachets	1, 2 and 2.4 g

Dose regimen:

Recommended starting dose in adults	7.2 g per day
Incremental doses	4.8 g every 3–4 days
Maintenance dose	Dependent on individual response
Maximum dose	24 g per day
Decremental doses	As for incremental doses in reverse

When high doses are used, an attempt should be made to reduce the dose of other AEDs.

Usual dose intervals: Two to three divided doses.

Serum level monitoring: Not useful.

Main side effects: Dizziness, insomnia, nausea, diarrhoea, weight gain, somnolence, depression, hypokinesia, rash.

Method of excretion: Renal.

Important interactions: Most anti-epileptic medication, oral contraceptives.

Teratogenic effects: Insufficient information because of restricted use.

Primidone

Brand names: Mysoline, Prominal.

Licensed in 1952 for all types of seizures except absence, for use in adults and children. This drug is now rarely prescribed for newly diagnosed patients. Some effort has been made to withdraw patients from this drug because of the long-term side effects, although withdrawal needs to be done over many months. This is not always successful because of the phenobarbitone content. Also, patients who are seizure-free are reluctant to risk the loss of control.

Because of the low cost, this drug, along with phenobarbitone, is still widely used in the developing world.

Usual preparations:

Tablets	30, 60, 200, 250 mg
Suspension:	250 mg / 5 ml (no longer listed in *BNF*, March 2001)

Dose regimen:

Recommended starting dose in adults and children	125 mg daily
Incremental doses	120–250 mg every 2 weeks
Maintenance dose in adults	500–1500 mg daily
Maintenance dose in children under 2 years	250–500 mg daily
Maintenance dose in children 2–5 years	500–750 mg daily
Maintenance dose in children 6–9 years	750–1000 mg daily
Maximum dose	Dependent on age or maximum tolerated dose
Decremental doses	Reduction will need to be very slow, depending on the length of time the person has been on the drug. Reductions may only be possible at 3-monthly intervals

Usual dose intervals: In adults and children, one to two divided doses per day.

Serum level monitoring: Not often used; is measured as phenobarbitone.

Target range: Check local normal values (e.g. 40–70 mmol/l phenobarbitone)

Main side effects: Acute dizziness, mood changes, aggression, cognitive dysfunction, dizziness, nausea, sedation, insomnia, hyperkinesis, impotence, reduced libido, folate deficiency, vitamin K and D deficiency, osteomalacia, rash, connective tissue abnormality, frozen shoulder.

Method of excretion: Hepatic.

Important interactions: Most anti-epileptic medication, oral contraceptives.

Teratogenic effects: Insufficient information because of limited use.

Tiagabine

Brand name: Gabitril.

Licensed in the UK in 1994. Used as add-on therapy for partial seizures with or without secondary generalization. Licensed for children over 12 years of age.

Usual preparations:

Tablets	5, 10, 15 mg

Dose regimen:

Recommended starting dose	5 mg daily
Incremental doses	5–10 mg weekly
Maintenance dose in adults (if added to enzyme-inducing drugs)	30–40 mg
Maintenance dose in adults (if added to non-enzyme inducing drugs)	15–30 mg
Maximum dose	15–30 mg daily
Decremental doses	As for incremental doses in reverse

Usual dose intervals: In adults and children, one to two divided doses if under 30 mg daily: three divided doses if over 30 mg daily.

Serum level monitoring: Not useful.

Main side effects: Diarrhoea, dizziness, tiredness, nervousness, tremor, emotional liability, speech impairment, concentration difficulties, depression, drowsiness, psychosis, rarely confusion, leucopenia.

Method of excretion: Hepatic.

Important interactions: Levels lowered when added to liver enzyme-inducing drugs (carbamazepine, phenytoin).

Teratogenic effects: Not known because of insufficient use.

Topiramate

Brand name: Topamax.

Licensed in the UK in 1994. Used as add-on therapy for partial seizures with or without secondary generalization, primary generalized seizures and Lennox–Gastaut syndrome. Licensed for children over 2 years of age.

Usual preparations:

Tablets	25, 50, 100, 200 mg
Sprinkle preparation	15, 25 mg

Dose regimen:

Recommended starting dose in adults	25–50 mg daily
Recommended starting dose in children	0.5 mg/kg daily
Incremental doses in adults	25–50 mg every 2 weeks
Incremental doses in children	1–3 mg/kg every 1–2 weeks
Maintenance dose in adults	200–600 mg daily
Maintenance dose in children	5–9 mg/kg daily
Maximum dose in adults	800 mg
Maximum dose in children	11 mg/kg
Decremental doses	As for incremental doses in reverse

Usual dose intervals: In adults and children, two divided doses.

Serum level monitoring: Not useful.

Main side effects: Abdominal pain, nausea, anorexia, weight loss, impaired concentration and memory, confusion, impaired speech, emotional lability, mood disorders, depression, altered behaviour, ataxia, abnormal gait, paraesthesia, dizziness, drowsiness, diplopia, nystagmus, taste disorder, psychosis, aggression, cognitive impairment, leucopenia.

Method of excretion: Renal.

Important interactions: Oral contraceptives.

Teratogenic effects: Not known because of insufficient use.

Sodium valproate

Brand names: Epilim, Epilim chrono, Convulex.

Licensed in 1973 (valproate acid licensed in 1993) as add-on or monotherapy for the use of all types of partial and primary generalized seizures including myoclonus. Also used for Lennox–Gastaut syndrome, childhood epilepsy syndromes and febrile convulsions. Because of the high risk of teratogenic effects and the possible increased incidence of polycystic ovary syndrome, this drug is now considered best avoided in young females and those of childbearing age, where possible. If this is the best drug of choice for the patient's seizure type, then specific advice is needed about planning pregnancies.

Usual preparations:

Enteric coated tablets	200, 500 mg
Crushable tablets	100 mg
Capsules	150, 300, 500 mg
Syrup	200 mg/5 ml
Liquid	200 mg/5 ml
Slow-release tablets	200, 300, 500 mg
Injection, powder for reconstitution	400 mg vial (mixed with 4 ml of water for injection)

The slow-release preparation is not suitable for children.

Dose regimen:

Recommended starting dose in adults	400–500 mg daily
Recommended starting dose in children under 20 kg	20 mg/kg daily
Recommended starting dose in children over 20 kg	40 mg/kg daily
Incremental doses in adults	200 mg every 1 week
Incremental doses in children	Increased slowly depending on clinical response, serum levels and chemical and haematological monitoring
Maintenance dose in adults	500–2500 mg daily
Maintenance dose in children under 20 kg	20–40 mg/kg daily
Maintenance dose in children over 20 kg	20–30 mg/kg daily

Maximum dose in adults	2500 mg daily
Maximum dose in children under 20 kg	35 mg/kg daily
Decremental doses	As for incremental doses in reverse

Intravenous regimen:

Initiating therapy	Intravenous injection over 3–5 minutes
In adults	400–800 mg/kg up to 10 mg/kg, followed by intravenous infusion up to 2.5 g daily
In children	Usually 20–30 mg/kg daily
When established oral therapy cannot be taken	Intravenous injection over 3–5 minutes or by intravenous infusion, continuing current oral dosage

Usual dose intervals: In adults and children, two to three divided doses daily.

Serum level monitoring: Not generally useful.

Target range: Check local values (recognized range 300–600 mmol/l).

Main side effects: Nausea, vomiting, gastric irritation, ataxia, tremor, increased appetite, weight gain, transient hair loss, oedema, thrombocytopenia, aggression, acute abdominal pain, pancreatitis, weakness, neutropenia, encepholopathy, irregular periods, amenorrhoea, hearing loss, dementia, Stevens–Johnson syndrome, vasculitis.

Method of excretion: Hepatic.

Important interactions: Interacts with many other AEDs. Dose adjustment needed when used in conjunction with lamotrigine.

Teratogenic effects: Increased incidence of spina bifida, foetal valproate syndrome, possibly increased incidence of learning difficulties in children exposed to valproate *in utero*.

Vigabatrin

Brand name: Sabril.

Licensed in 1989 as add-on therapy for adults and children for all types of seizures not controlled on first-line drugs. Now licensed as monotherapy in children with West's syndrome (infantile spasms) and Lennox–Gastaut syndrome. Rarely used now in adults because of problems with visual field defects.

Usual preparations:

Tablets	500 mg
Powder sachet	500 mg

Dose regimen:

Recommended starting dose in adults	1000 mg daily
Recommended starting dose in children	40 mg/kg daily, or 500–1000 mg daily (bodyweight 10–15 kg) or 1500–3000 mg daily (body weight over 30 kg)
Incremental doses in adults	500 mg every week
Incremental doses in children	Dependent on clinical response
Maintenance dose in adults	2–4 g daily
Maintenance dose in children	80–100 mg/kg daily, or 500 mg–1 g daily (body weight 10–15 kg), or 1 g–1.5 g daily (body weight 15–30 kg), or 1.5–3 g daily (body weight 30–50 kg, or 2–4 g daily (body weight over 50 kg)
Maximum dose in adults	6 g daily
Maximum dose in children	11 mg/kg
Decremental doses	As for incremental doses in reverse

Dose when used as monotherapy for West's syndrome: 60–100 mg/kg daily adjusting over 7 days up to 150 mg/kg daily depending on tolerance. It is usually well tolerated.

Usual dose intervals: In adults and children, one to two divided doses daily.

Serum level monitoring: Not useful.

Main side effects: Irreversible severe visual field constriction, sedation, dizziness, headache, ataxia, paraesthesia, agitation, amnesia, mood changes, depression, psychosis, aggression, confusion, weight gain, tremor, diplopia, diarrhoea, drowsiness, fatigue, nervousness, irritability, agitation, abnormal thinking, headache, nystagmus, ataxia, tremor, impaired concentration, mania, memory disturbance, increased seizure frequency.

Method of excretion: Renal.

Contraindications: In some patients behavioural changes have been seen; it is not recommended in patients with a history of psychosis or behavioural problems.

This drug may also cause problems in patients with a history of renal impairment. These patients should be monitored for signs of any problems.

Important interactions: Vigabatrin may lower phenytoin levels.

Teratogenic effect: Because this is a relatively new drug there is little information available. However, it is not recommended in pregnancy, as there were teratogenic effects in animals during the trial period.

Additional drugs used in the treatment of epilepsy

Acetazolamide (Diamox, Diamox SR)

Acetazolamide is a second-line drug for tonic–clonic and partial seizures. It is occasionally helpful in atypical absence, atonic and tonic seizures. The usual dose is 250 mg one to three times daily. Tolerance may develop with continuous use over 3–6 months. Withdrawal and reintroduction can regain effectiveness.

Benzodiazepines

Diazepam (Valium): Used as an emergency drug in the treatment of prolonged seizures and status epilepticus. Can be given as oral, rectal or intravenous preparation. The dose regimen will depend on the situation in which it is being used, and it is given according to the patient's weight. Rectal diazepam is often used in children or in people with a learning disability, where prolonged seizures may be a recurring problem. Because of the problems with respiratory depression associated with this drug, dosing and frequency of use need to be monitored carefully. Intravenous administration is generally only used in hospital situation; the patient should have cardiac monitoring during this procedure. If prescribed for rectal administration individual protocols should be initiated.

Midazolam: Owing to the difficulties of administering rectal diazepam (particularly in a public place) experimental usage has been made of midazolam by the buccal and intra-nasal routes. These options sound very promising, but have yet to be fully evaluated and are not licensed for this method of use.

Clonazepam (Rivotril): This is used as adjunctive therapy in partial and generalized seizures, including absence seizures, myoclonus and Lennox–Gastaut syndrome. It is usually added when all other drugs have failed. Tolerance to this drug may develop in a few months in some patients, so rendering it ineffective.

Usual preparations:

Tablets	0.5, 2 mg
Liquid	1 mg in 1 ml

Dose regimen: 0.5 mg daily increasing to 4 mg daily (in divided doses).

Clobazam Frisium: This is used as adjunctive therapy for partial and generalized seizures, and often as intermittent therapy in the treatment of cluster seizures, in the treatment of non-convulsive status epilepticus, or in situations where extra cover is needed for a short period of time.

Preparation: Tablets, capsules 10 mg.

Dose regimen: 10–30 mg daily. This drug is sometimes used on an intermittent basis, e.g. in hormone-related epilepsy.

The following applies to all drugs in the benzodiazepine category:

Side effects: Drowsiness, sedation, fatigue, ataxia, dizziness, restlessness, irritability, aggression, behavioural disturbance.

Use with caution in patients with respiratory, hepatic and renal disease. Respiratory depression may occur if it is given in too high a dose intravenously.

> Remember that people who have epilepsy requiring continuous anticonvulsant therapy can get exemption from prescription charges. They can apply for this on form P11 from the DSS Office, doctor's surgery or chemist.

Withdrawing anticonvulsant therapy

It is important to remember that anticonvulsant therapy should never be stopped suddenly. Even if a drug is thought to have been ineffective in controlling seizures, this practice may lead to a sudden increase in seizure activity.

When changes of medication are being made to improve seizure control:

- The new drug should be introduced up to a therapeutic dose before any other drugs are withdrawn, or
- The drug being introduced and the one being withdrawn need to be carefully titrated in equal doses
- Drugs such as phenytoin and phenobarbitone need to be withdrawn very slowly following prolonged use to avoid rebound seizures – e.g. phenytoin 25 mg every 4–8 weeks; phenobarbitone 15–30 mg every 1–3 months depending on the duration of therapy prior to withdrawal.

The initial stages of withdrawal may be undertaken with no problems, but the later stages still need close monitoring because this is when problems may occur. In some cases it may not be possible to undertake total withdrawal of the medication and maintain seizure control.

The specialist nurse can help to establish a plan for these actions.

Patients who have become seizure-free

In these cases, careful consideration should be given to the following situations. These may act as predictors for the risk of seizures recurring:

- Any known reasons for the condition occurring, e.g. known underlying structural lesion found at diagnosis
- Past medical history, e.g. febrile convulsions
- The type of epilepsy, e.g. myoclonic/photosensitive; these may carry up to a 90 per cent risk of seizures recurring
- The age of onset of the epilepsy
- How quickly seizures were controlled following the start of medication.

It is also important to bear in mind the social implications for the person if seizures recur following withdrawal – e.g. the possible loss of a driving licence.

Dose withdrawal

For most drugs, the recommended plan for withdrawal would be to reverse the regime by which the drug was introduced.

If the patient has developed a reaction to a drug and a more rapid withdrawal is needed, then advice should be sought from a neurologist or the prescribing consultant. This is important, as an alternative drug may need to be substituted to maintain seizure control.

Summary of need to monitor anti-epileptic drug serum levels

Monitoring of almost any AED is available, but many would have to be sent to specialized laboratories. However, for most newer AEDs and some older ones there is no close connection between serum levels and anticonvulsant effect, so measuring serum levels does not aid in monitoring the effectiveness of drug therapy.

Reliability of results: Individual reactions to drugs vary and are not always related to the measurable therapeutic levels. For example:

- Some patients will need to maintain a higher than recommended serum level to obtain optimal control and have no side effects, while others will have optimal control at a virtually sub-therapeutic level.
- Some patients will have signs of toxicity at very low dosage levels; this may occur when medication is first commenced if initial dosing is too high, or when the dose is being increased too quickly.
- Some drug interaction will result in increased retention of metabolites with normal serum levels, resulting in inappropriate management of drug changes (e.g. lamotrigine and carbamazepine).

Trough levels are not always an accurate guide to dose adjustment – with carbamazepine, the difference between trough and peak may vary greatly.

In general, serum concentrations do not contribute greatly to defining the optimal dose of a particular AED for an individual patient; this is better done by clinical assessment.

People metabolize drugs at different rates, and therefore the optimum dose for one may result in poor control or toxicity in another. This will also affect peak trough differentials and the interpretation of these.

Routine 'prophylactic' monitoring: Routine measuring of serum AED concentrations in patients who are well controlled and not experiencing unwanted effects is not necessary. In the absence of clinical concern, this needs to be done no more than every 12–24 months and only in a few drugs (e.g. carbamazepine and phenytoin). Routine testing may lead to inappropriate and unnecessary changes being made, leading to loss of control or the onset of side effects.

Special categories of patients:
- Acutely unwell patients may need monitoring every 24 hours or more frequently (patients in this category will usually be hospitalized if this is necessary).
- Pregnant patients will need monitoring during steady state prior to conception, and during the first and last trimesters to determine any changes in serum levels due to changes in the disposition of the drug in pregnancy.
- People with learning disability – it is more important to monitor this group, but the need should still relate to the patient's clinical state. As much assessment as possible should still relate to patient's ability to report problems. Others can record increased seizures. Possible unwanted effects need to be assessed by direct questions worded at a level the patient can understand. Some behavioural changes may be related to unwanted effects (e.g. head rubbing may indicate headache or double vision).

Limitations of the utility of therapeutic range of AEDs:
- The concept of the therapeutic 'target ranges' of serum concentrations of AEDs is often abused. The quoted ranges should simply be given as indications of the concentrations at which the majority of patients have optimum seizure control, and above which dose-related effects are more likely to occur.
- Zealous adherence to quoted ranges is inappropriate and AED concentration data should always be subject to, and interpreted in, the light of clinical data.
- Approximately 20 per cent of patients attending a London clinic have optimal control with serum AED concentrations outside quoted ranges.

Conclusions

The monitoring of AED levels may be relevant to patient care. It is however important to remember that serum levels need to be taken in context with clinical data obtained.

- Patients having no adverse effects from AEDs and good

seizure control are on a high enough dose of drug, whatever that may be.

- In patients having adverse effects that are dose-related, a dose reduction should be considered whatever the original dose.
- In patients continuing to have seizures, an increased dose should be considered up to maximum level as long as no unwanted effects occur.
- If seizures continue at the maximum recommended or tolerated dosage, a drug change needs to be considered – either the substitution of an alternative first-line drug, or the addition of a second-line drug.

SURGICAL TREATMENT OF EPILEPSY

Surgical treatment for epilepsy was first reported in 1880. The procedure has continued to develop with the improvements in anaesthesia and surgical techniques. The outcomes following surgery have improved with the better understanding of epilepsy and the advances in investigations and assessment processes available. The introduction of magnetic resonance imaging (MRI) has been a major factor in the increase in the use of resectional surgery.

Surgical treatment for epilepsy can be divided into three categories:

1. Surgery for the treatment of underlying structural lesions such as cerebral tumours or vascular lesions
2. Resectional surgery carried out specifically to reduce seizure frequency
3. The fitting of vagal nerve stimulators.

Surgery for underlying pathology

Cerebral tumours

Epilepsy occurs in approximately 50 per cent of patients with intracranial tumours, although the incidence will vary depending on the type and position of the tumour. Table 8.5 shows the approximate incidence of epilepsy associated with different tumour types.

Table 8.5 The incidence of epilepsy associated with different tumour types

Tumour type	Approximate incidence of seizures (%)
Acute onset epilepsy:	
Oligodendrogliomas	92
Astocytomas	70
Glioblastomas	37
Chronic refractory epilepsy:	
Oligodendrogliomas	10–30
Dysembryoplastic neuroepithelial	10–30
Gangliomas	10–20
Hamartomas	10–20

Slow-growing or benign tumours are the cause of epilepsy in approximately 10 per cent of adults and less than 10 per cent of children with the condition. The history of epilepsy may have been present for many years – even decades – before the tumour is identified.

The surgical outcome will depend on the tumour type, although where the tumour is slow growing and can be completely removed, approximately 70–90 per cent of patients will be seizure-free after surgery. Where partial resection is undertaken or surrounding tissue is removed, then the epilepsy may not be controlled or residual effects will present.

Other underlying causes of epilepsy

Underlying cause	Association with chronic epilepsy
Arteriovenous malformation	20–40%
Cortical dysgenesis	15–20%
Cerebral infection	Dependent on the sight of infection
Trauma	Dependent on the type of trauma

Surgery carried out specifically to reduce seizure frequency

1. Focal resection for hippocampal sclerosis:
   - temporal lobectomy

- amygdalohippocampectomy.
2. Focal resection for other lesions:
   - lesionectomy in temporal lobe
   - lesionectomy in other lobes.
3. Non-lesional focal resection:
   - frontal lobectomy
   - other restricted resections.
4. Multilobar resection:
   - hemispherectomy
   - other multilobar resections.
5. Functional procedures:
   - corpus callosectomy
   - multiple subpial transection
   - vagal nerve stimulation
   - stereotactic stimulation.

Surgical treatment of temporal lobe epilepsy

The most common of these procedures is resection for hippocampal sclerosis causing temporal lobe epilepsy. In this procedure a variable amount of the temporal lobe is removed. Generally less is taken on the dominant (usually left) side, as the left posterior temporal lobe is closely associated with language centres.

Most patients referred for consideration of surgery are those with a diagnosis of chronic intractable epilepsy where it is not possible to achieve control without unacceptable side effects from the medication. This is because of the risks associated with the surgery and the possible post-operative complications (see Table 8.6).

Where preoperative evaluation has been carefully undertaken prior to temporal lobectomy:

- 60–70 per cent of patients will be seizure-free
- 20 per cent will have significant seizure reduction
- 10–20 per cent will experience no change.

Seizure frequency at 1 year post-surgery can be used as a reliable predictor of long-term outcomes:

- If seizures continue, there is < 10 per cent incidence of remission over the next 5 years

Table 8.6 Post-operative complications following surgical treatment for temporal lobe epilepsy

Complication	Approximate incidence
Homonymous visual field defect	20%
Complete hemianopia	35%
Hemiplegia	1%
Transient mild dysphasia	Common when dominant lobe is resected
Permanent dysphasia	<1%
Permanent dysphasia	<1%
Mild memory/intellectual deficit	Rare, may improve after surgery
Profound amnesia	Rare
Psychiatric disturbance	15% (usually transient)
Permanent psychotic breakdown	<5%
Depression	Common in first year
Serious permanent complications (including third nerve palsy, meningitis, scalp infection, subdural haematoma/empyema, hydrocephalus)	<5%
Mortality	<0.5%

- If the patient is seizure-free, there is <10 per cent incidence of relapse over next 5 years.

Medication following surgery

When patients are seizure-free following surgery, medication is usually continued unchanged for 12–24 months, and then for a further 12 months at a reduced dose.

When seizures continue following surgery, regular follow-up and adjustment of medication will continue to obtain the best level of control possible.

Counselling and support

This will be essential where seizures continue following surgery.

Counselling and support will also be necessary for patients attaining a seizure-free state, as some problems associated with epilepsy will not be resolved by removing the seizures. There will need to be a time of adjustment, which will vary depending on the age of onset of the epilepsy and the age at which surgery is undertaken. The person may need to learn to develop inter-personal skills or may have missed educational opportunities, resulting in difficulty in obtaining employment when the epilepsy is controlled. For some the loss of benefits that may accompany seizure freedom may result in financial difficulties, resulting in new problems.

Post-traumatic epilepsy

- Head injuries following road traffic accident, falls or recreational injuries account for about 2–12 per cent of all cases of epilepsy
- Mild head injuries (no fracture and less than 30 minutes post-traumatic amnesia) give no increased risk of epilepsy
- Moderate head injuries (skull fracture plus more than 30 minutes post-traumatic amnesia) give a 1–2 per cent risk of epilepsy
- Severe head injuries (intracranial haematoma or cerebral contusion plus more than 24 hours amnesia) give a 10 per cent risk of epilepsy
- Following open or penetrating head injury, the incidence of epilepsy is 50 per cent.

Epilepsy following neurosurgical procedures

We have discussed ways in which surgery can be used to treat epilepsy; however, it is important to remember that for many undergoing a neurosurgical procedure may result in the onset of seizures. In this section we will discuss the incidence of epilepsy following neurosurgical conditions.

Epilepsy after neurosurgery

Shorvon (2000) studied 877 patients with no previous history of seizures who had surgery for non-traumatic conditions. Patients were followed up for 5 years and the following outcomes recorded:

Surgery	Incidence of epilepsy (%)
Stereotactic surgery	4
Craniotomy for glioma	19
Intracranial haemorrhage	21
Removal of meningioma	22
Treatment for cerebral abscess	92
Following shunt procedures	10

Thirty-seven per cent of seizures occurred within 1 year of surgery, and 92% occurred within 2 years.

Surgery for treatment of aneurysm:

Surgery	Incidence of epilepsy (%)
Unruptured aneurysm	14
Middle cerebral aneurysm	19
Posterior communicating aneurysm	10

If there has been an intracranial haematoma, the incidence may be higher.

Vagal nerve stimulation

This method of treatment was approved in the USA in 1998, and is used in patients with chronic refractory epilepsy. The procedure involves fitting a stimulator in the chest cavity with an electrode connected to the left vagal nerve. The stimulator is adjusted according to individuals' needs by use of a magnet. Patients can also use a magnet to activate additional stimuli in between the pre-set rate. Clinical trials have been carried out on patients between the ages of 13 and 60 years with different seizure types; three levels of stimulation were used.

Opinions vary as to the potential value of vagal nerve stimulation as a form of treatment. Some results seem to indicate that the effect on seizure control is minimal, although there have also been reports of good response in seizure reduction in children in some American studies (Fisher *et al.*, 1999). Because this is still a relatively new method of treatment, it is difficult to estimate its potential use in the future.

The procedure is not without side effects, including:

- Alteration of voice
- Dyspnoea
- A tingling feeling in the neck with each stimulation.

ADDITIONAL FORMS OF TREATMENT

One of the main problems with a diagnosis of epilepsy is that the person with the condition often feels out of control. We have discussed medical and surgical treatments for epilepsy; in this section we will discuss additional forms of treatment that may help the person to feel more in control. These treatments will not replace the medication, but in some cases may result in lower doses being required.

Often people with epilepsy are told that massage and other complementary therapies are not safe. This is usually not true, although any form of complementary therapy should only be undertaken under the supervision of a qualified therapist.

Avoidance technique

If a person has only ever had a seizure when put into a particular situation, then avoiding that situation is an important factor for controlling the seizures. Examples include:

- Being sensitive to flashing lights
- Being sensitive to particular patterns, or styles of writing
- Being sensitive to certain colour combinations
- Not having enough sleep
- Getting too worried or excited
- Getting an infection and a high temperature (not a febrile convulsion, which is different).

It must be remembered that most people will not be able to find a trigger for their seizures, but if they can, then it will help to improve control. If the patient keeps a record of the seizures and what happens before, during and after them, this will help in identifying any triggers.

Some people will find that by learning to concentrate on a particular picture, piece of music or smell, they can overcome a seizure. This method can only be effective if there is some warning that a seizure is going to occur. If they are taught self-hypnosis to use in conjunction with their chosen method, this can become very effective for a few people.

Areas of complementary therapy that may be helpful include:

- Relaxation
- Massage
- Yoga
- Hypnosis.

Aromatherapy may also help, but care must be taken in choosing oils:

Oils that may be helpful	Oils to be avoided
Ylang Ylang	Rosemary
Camomile	Hyssop
Lavender	Sweet fennel
Jasmine	Sage

Recently, the potential problem associated with the use of St John's Wort for depression received prominence. It was reported that St John's Wort may have an effect on the serum levels of some anti-epileptic medications, thereby increasing the risk of seizures.

Depression and many of the recognized antidepressant drugs can also affect seizure control, and may be more problematic than St John's Wort. Any people with epilepsy taking St John's Wort should not suddenly stop using it; they should however be advised that this preparation does interact with the oral contraceptive pill and will reduce its effectiveness.

9 Children with epilepsy

INTRODUCTION

Although the basic concepts of epilepsy and medication have been covered in previous sections, here we will be looking at specific issues relating to children and adolescents. There are many causes and presentations that may differ from those seen in adults; there are also additional differential diagnoses to be considered.

Seizures are more common in children than adults, but not all seizures are epilepsy. This does not mean that they are any less frightening to the parents, and a great deal of support will be needed whatever the cause.

Between 5 and 6 per cent of children will have some form of attack that will lead to altered consciousness or convulsions, and most of these will not be due to epilepsy. The prevalence of epilepsy is about four per 1000 (0.4 per cent).

Owing to the immaturity of the cortex and white matter tracts in the child's brain, the presentation of epilepsy may be different from that seen in adults. As the child grows and the brain continues to develop, the clinical features of a seizure may change. This may lead to the misunderstanding that the nature or classification has changed, but this is not the case. It may only be possible to establish a clear classification and prognosis as the child gets older. Appropriate treatment may not always be easily identified until this later stage of development.

GETTING THE DIAGNOSIS RIGHT

Although paediatricians emphasize that children are not small adults and may have different presentation of the seizures, there are common factors when it comes to making the correct diagnosis:

- Performing a basic medical examination to establish general health.
- Obtaining a description of the episode from a witness and, where possible, the child. Where the witness has been a teacher or carer, ask the family to obtain a written description; this will be essential when referring the child to a specialist.
- Establishing any possible trigger factors (e.g. fever, infection).
- Considering other causes of loss of consciousness.

In a child or adolescent, obtaining a developmental history may be more important than where epilepsy presents in an adults.

Differential diagnosis

Paediatric neurologists found that 10–30 per cent of children referred to specialist clinics with poorly controlled epilepsy did not in fact have the condition.

The most commonly mistaken conditions are:

- Anoxic seizure
- Sleep disturbances in young children
- Syncope in adolescents.

FEBRILE CONVULSIONS

Febrile convulsions are not always considered to be a form of epilepsy but are symptomatic seizures; it is important to discuss the implications of these seizures in children, because they are a major cause of concern for the family.

These type of seizures may occur in between 3 and 5 per cent of children up to the age of 6 years. Many will have only one episode. Most febrile seizures will be generalized, self-limiting and usually brief. They are more common in male infants or in those where there is a family history of febrile convulsions and epilepsy. Most children will have only one seizure, although

30–50 per cent may have a second and 10 per cent may have three or more seizures.

The approximate incidence and age-related presentation of seizures is shown in Table 9.1.

Table 9.1 Incidence and age-related presentation of febrile convulsions

Incidence (%)	Age
4	<6 months
50	in the second year
90	in the first 3 years
6	>6 years

Eighty per cent of the seizures are caused by viral infection, and 8 per cent by viral or bacterial meningitis.

Actions to be taken when a seizure occurs

- First aid during these seizures is the same as in any other generalized seizure
- Examination should be undertaken to exclude serious underlying causes (e.g. meningitis)
- If no cause is found, then the appropriate treatment is to cool the child and administer a paracetamol preparation to prevent further spikes in temperature
- If the seizure lasts for more than 5 minutes, rectal diazepam 5–10 mg may be given (dosing will depend on the child's age and weight).

Admission to hospital is advisable following a first seizure to establish a possible underlying cause, but may not always be necessary with subsequent seizures if correct advice and support is given to the parents.

Prolonged seizures (those lasting for 15 minutes or longer) will always need emergency treatment.

Between 6 and 18 per cent of children having these seizures may develop a learning disability, although the seizures are probably not the cause but occur because of existing cerebral damage resulting in a lowered threshold to seizures.

Approximately 10 per cent of children experiencing febrile seizures lasting for more than 30 minutes, or presenting with focal signs, may develop temporal lobe epilepsy with clinical evidence of temporal lobe damage on imaging. The epilepsy may not present until the child is between 6 years and adolescence. The link between temporal lobe epilepsy and febrile seizures has been raised, although this type of epilepsy is seen in adolescence with no history of febrile convulsions and no evidence of structural damage on imaging. Because of this uncertainty it is important to ensure the correct treatment of febrile seizures to reduce the risk of potential long-term implications.

CONSIDERING DIFFERENT AGE GROUPS

Seizures occurring in the neonatal period are usually related to underlying structural or metabolic causes, e.g. hypoglycaemia, cerebral malformation, birth anoxia, drug withdrawal from maternal medication etc. Where seizures do occur in this age group, they are usually symptomatic and often related to some form of syndrome (e.g. West syndrome – infantile spasm).

Many seizures occurring following the neonatal period will not be epilepsy. The developing brain is very susceptible to outside influences, the most common of these being fever. As the child grows the continuing development of the brain means that seizure presentation may be more defined. However, this does not necessarily make diagnosis easier.

Twenty-five per cent of all seizures presenting in older children are thought to be benign partial seizures. They seem to be more common in boys than girls, and include symptoms such as unilateral paraesthesia of the tongue, lips and cheek. They may also present as a unilateral clonic convulsion involving the face, lips, tongue and larynx. In these speech may be affected although there is no loss of consciousness. This may not be recognized, as the child's inability to respond may be mistaken for a disturbance in the conscious level. Attacks most commonly occur on waking, and the child may also have tonic–clonic seizures. In most cases diagnosis can be confirmed by the EEG findings. Prognosis is good, treatment is effective, and the seizures almost always stop at puberty.

Diagnosis may be difficult when a child presents with absence attacks. These may be diagnosed as childhood absences (petit mal), as this is often thought to be the only presentation of this type of seizure in this age group. Consideration should always be given to the possibility that these may be complex partial absences.

To help distinguish the difference between these seizures:

1. *Childhood absences* are almost always brief, rarely lasting more than 30 seconds, and are usually associated with eyelid fluttering. Occasionally these may present in a modified form with some mild automatisms in longer attacks. Recovery is immediate, with the child able to continue any previous actions without delay.
2. In *complex partial seizures* the attack will be longer lasting, and any automatism will be more pronounced than in childhood absences. Recovery will take longer, and the child may be confused afterwards, not remembering his or her actions prior to the episode. Differentiating these attacks is important, because the treatment and prognosis are different. An EEG will usually help differentiate between the two types of childhood absences.

Tonic–clonic seizures will not always be primary generalized, although the child may not readily acknowledge any warning of the seizures. With careful history taking it may be possible to identify a warning experienced by the child, although it may not always be possible to establish a focus on investigation. These may be identified as cryptogenic epilepsy.

Partial seizures do occur in childhood, and are usually symptomatic in origin. For children over 10 years of age absence seizures will almost certainly be partial, as true childhood absence 'petit mal' rarely present after this age.

The prognosis for most seizure types occurring in childhood or adolescence is good unless the seizures are associated with an underlying structural lesion.

Where a child has presented with seizures at an early age, the presence of a definable syndrome may become more apparent as he or she grows. Definition of different seizure types in one child will play an important part in establishing the presence of a syndrome. We will not discuss syndromes at this point, although they include:

- West syndrome
- Lenoux–Gastoux syndrome
- Sturge–Weber syndrome
- Tubersclerosis.

As the child approaches adolescence, the presentation of the seizure may vary from that when the child was younger. This will help with establishing a diagnosis if this has not been possible in the past. It is important periodically to update seizure descriptions as the child grows, particularly where a diagnosis has not been established.

SEIZURE TYPES

These are discussed fully in Chapter 6, and are briefly reviewed in this section.

1. *Generalized seizures* include:
   - absence seizures
   - photosensitive seizures, which may present as absence or tonic–clonic seizures
   - drop attacks
   - atonic and tonic seizures.
2. *Partial seizures* may be symptomatic, especially if associated with localizing signs, and include:
   - temporal lobe seizures – some presentations may be confused with generalized infantile absence seizures
   - frontal lobe seizures, which may be confused with night terrors or bizarre behaviour
   - occipital lobe seizures, which may be confused with migraine
   - benign rolandic epilepsy, which is non-symptomatic and is diagnosed by typical EEG findings.
3. *Juvenile myoclonic seizures* – only about 10 per cent of patients will remit; the rest may need lifelong medication even if they

become seizure-free. Often the child presents following a generalized early morning seizure. It is important to determine whether there has been a history of early morning clumsiness prior to this seizure.

Early correct classification is important to help with prognosis and management.

Education may become a problem because of increasing numbers of seizure or difficulties with medication. There may be absence seizures, and the memory may be affected if seizures are not controlled.

Temporal lobe epilepsy is often the most suitable for surgical treatment. If there is no response to drugs, surgery may also be considered for some children with temporal or frontal lobe seizures, particularly if these are post-traumatic in origin.

TREATMENT

It is important to remember that medication should not be commenced until there is a definite diagnosis. At present it is not common practice to commence treatment at any age following a single seizure. If a child is continuing to have seizures between the referral and the appointment, then it is important to seek advice from the paediatric department where the referral has been made. If possible, a clear description of the seizure should be taken and documented at the time of presentation to the GP surgery (memories change over time).

Correct diagnosis and seizure typing are essential to allow a prognosis to be given. This will avoid inappropriate withdrawal of medication and its consequences, or unnecessary continuation of long-term treatment.

Misdiagnosis may also affect future prospects, as some careers are barred to anyone having had a diagnosis of epilepsy – even if they become seizure-free.

When implementing medication, the following factors should be considered:

- The type of epilepsy
- The child's age
- The preparations available

- The possible need for long-term medication
- Any co-morbidity.

When a decision has been made about the type of medication to be prescribed, then other factors that will need consideration are:

1. The increased metabolism in children.
2. The dosing regimes to be used – these can be problematic:
    - it may be necessary on occasions to administer drugs more frequently during the day than recommended by the manufacturers, in order to maintain adequate serum levels
    - frequent dosing during the day may cause problems with drug administration at school
    - frequent dosing during the day increases the risk of non-compliance because of forgotten midday doses
    - the more times the child has to take the medication, the greater the reinforcement of them 'being different'
    - many of the drugs are not licenced for or have not undergone adequate pharmacokinetic studies in children.
3. Drug interactions, current or future (oral contraception).
4. Pregnancy issues – these may need to be considered even in childhood.

The latter two are important even with young children, as advice will need to be given early if future problems are to be avoided. Children become sexually active at an age that may appear surprisingly young to us wrinkly health care professionals, and even more so to their parents! This topic is usually difficult for children to talk about in the presence of their parents. The child may remain on medication but no longer be under regular review, so even if not sexually active at the time of the initial discussion, these issues will become important.

Specific information on individual drugs is covered in Chapter 7; information regarding sexuality and family planning is discussed in Chapter 9.

10 Sexuality and planning a family

SEXUALITY

Most people with epilepsy will have no problem with sexuality or forming relationships; for some, however, there may be a problem.

The issue of sexuality can be a problem for both men and women. For both sexes the possibility of overprotection and reduced contact with their peers as a child may lead to problems in forming relationships and sharing their feelings with others in later life. If the person's epilepsy is still active, there may also be the fear that a seizure will occur during sexual intercourse. If there is more input with the family and better understanding of the problems caused by overprotection of children, this may become less of a problem.

There is little evidence to show that women with epilepsy have sexually-related problems. Research undertaken has usually concentrated on trying to identify problems related to drug therapy and has been carried out in specialist epilepsy centres, and therefore may not be representative of the average person with epilepsy. There have been no direct comparison studies undertaken. The greatest problem appears to be that of possible reduced sexual drive and fertility because of the epilepsy itself rather than the medication.

Both sexes may have feelings of sexual arousal related to a partial seizure disorder; however, these are part of the seizure or of post-seizure confusion.

Studies undertaken by Morrell indicate that up to 50 per cent of men may have a problem with functional arousal rather than with the desire to have sex. This is not necessarily associated with reduced opportunity to have sex. There is often an inability to achieve or to maintain an erection. This appears to be more common in men with temporal lobe partial seizures arising from the amygdala and hippocampus, and where the epilepsy is uncontrolled. There is evidence of increased prolactin levels in men with epilepsy, whether they are on anticonvulsant medication or not. Raised prolactin levels are a known cause of impotence. There is no apparent evidence of sexual problems being related to the number of anticonvulsant drugs taken or the doses. Anecdotal evidence, however, does not always agree with this finding. When the epilepsy is treated either with medication or temporal lobe surgery, the sexually-related problems also improve.

FERTILITY

Fertility problems can arise in men and women with epilepsy, and these may be related to the epilepsy or the medication.

Women's issues

The impact of epilepsy and medication on the menstrual cycle

- Thirty-five per cent of women with temporal lobe epilepsy are likely to have menstrual problems, compared to 8 per cent of women who do not have epilepsy
- There may be a delay in the onset of menstruation in girls with epilepsy
- There is thought to be an increased incidence of polycystic ovary syndrome in women with epilepsy who are not on medication
- There is thought to be a greater increase in polycystic ovary syndrome in women taking sodium valproate
- There is some evidence of prolonged cycles and irregular menstruation, and there also may be an increased incidence of amenorrhoeas and oligomenorrhoeas in women on sodium valproate.

Men's issues

There is little research or evidence regarding infertility-related problems in men with epilepsy. Isojarvi and Morrell are undertaking research into possibly sexually-related disorders associated with epilepsy and anticonvulsant medication. As with women, much of the research has been undertaken in specialist units and residential care settings where results may not be truly representative. More research is currently being undertaken in the area.

The only definite evidence is that carbamazepine has been associated with impotence and impaired fertility (possibly a reduced sperm count). These problems appear to resolve when the drug is withdrawn.

CONTRACEPTION

The failure rate of the oral contraceptive may be as high as 7 per cent for any female. Drugs may have an impact on its efficiency, although women are often prescribed these without being advised about the interaction between the drug and the pill. Antibiotics are often prescribed without advice about drug interactions.

Women with epilepsy need specific advice about contraception, but there is no reason why they should not be prescribed an oral contraceptive if they are monitored correctly for breakthrough bleeding and have been informed of the risk of reduced effectiveness. Problems arise when the women are taking a liver enzyme-inducing drug such as:

- carbamazepine
- phenytoin
- topiramate
- primidone

or any of the barbiturates: these all increase the metabolism of oestrogen and progestogen. This makes progestogen-only pills unreliable and it is recommended that, if these are used, the dose be doubled. The depot progestogen injection should be administered every 10 weeks instead of every 12 weeks.

The same anti-epileptic drugs (AEDs) also affect the combined contraceptive pill. Recommendations for this type of pill are that a dose of at least 50 mg of oestrogen (e.g. Ovran) be given initially; the women should also be advised to use some form of barrier contraceptive until reliability has been established. If no breakthrough bleeding occurs, the pill can be considered as effective as possible. However, if breakthrough bleeding does occur, then initially the pack can be 'tricycled' (e.g. three packs taken in succession with a 4-day break before commencing the next set of packs). The woman should be informed that bleeding might continue for a few days after the next set of packs is started. If problems continue on this regimen, the dose can be adjusted by adding a 25-mg pill and, if necessary, a second 50-mg pill.

If absolute certainty about contraceptive control is needed, progesterone levels should be checked on the twenty-first day of the cycle.

Emergency contraception (oral hormonal method)

There are no specific recommendations for the use of emergency contraception where the woman is taking AEDs, although the *BNF* does recommend that the dose be increased by 50 per cent (to three tablets if the person is taking liver enzyme-inducing drugs; see p. 149).

> If you are not sure about the correct information on any of the above issues, please refer to the *British National Formulary* or contact your local epilepsy specialist nurse before giving any advice to a patient.
> If you do give advice, ensure that you check the patient's correct medication and possible interactions, and document any information given.

EPILEPSY AND PREGNANCY

> **Important**: It is unwise to make radical changes in anti-epileptic medication once a pregnancy has started. If a woman presents and is already pregnant, stopping the treatment to protect the foetus at this point is inappropriate. This will have no impact on any risk to the foetus, but may induce loss of control of the seizures.

When addressing issues regarding epilepsy and pregnancy, there are three broad areas to be considered:

1. Pre-conception
2. Pregnancy and delivery
3. Breast-feeding and baby care.

In addition, some women with epilepsy may need specific genetic counselling. This is a complex field, and is beyond the scope of this book.

It may be possible for much of this advice to be given by the same person, but if there is no individual professional with adequate training then the counselling and advice may be undertaken by different professionals. It is of course very important that the person providing this advice knows what he or she is talking about.

For pregnancies continuing to full term, there is more than a 90 per cent chance of an uneventful pregnancy resulting in a healthy baby.

Pre-pregnancy counselling

Initial advice regarding the risk to a pregnancy of medication or uncontrolled seizures should be given by the doctor when the diagnosis is made, and before medication is introduced. This will help the woman to make an informed choice about the risks she may be taking in later life. Up to half of pregnancies are unplanned, so planning for the eventuality should be an integral part of the information for any woman with childbearing potential who has epilepsy. An epilepsy specialist nurse may also have given the woman advice and information early in the diagnosis. Even where initial information has been given, women should still ideally be referred for further counselling when planning a pregnancy.

If there is no neurologist or epilepsy specialist nurse in your area, the necessary information and advice can be provided by a genetic counsellor, and advice regarding the risk from the drugs can be obtained from the local drug information department at the nearest hospital. If it is not possible to obtain any information locally, the British Epilepsy Association is able to provide advice about the nearest specialist nurse who may be able to help.

When undertaking pre-pregnancy counselling, it is important to establish whether any initial counselling and advice have been given. If so the subject should still be discussed; it may be that incomplete information was given initially, or that new information is currently available.

It is important not only to concentrate on the information associated with the epilepsy and medication but also on any family history of neural tube defects, cardiac defects or auro-facial defects. These will be important when assessing potential risk factors.

All women with epilepsy should be prescribed 5 mg folic acid daily for a minimum of 3 months prior to conception. This should be continued at least until the end of the first trimester, although some units recommend that this it be continued throughout the pregnancy.

It is important to be sure that all the facts are discussed so that a woman can make an informed choice about whether to continue on medication or even whether to change the drug. This should include the risks not only of the medication but also of uncontrolled seizures. Consideration will need to be taken of the type of epilepsy and the length of time taken to obtain seizure control. The seizure type will also be relevant. A simple partial seizure may cause no problem, whereas a tonic–clonic seizure could be dangerous to both mother and baby.

Depending on local protocol, if the women is seizure-free and on medication it may be appropriate to measure drug serum levels at this stage to establish her appropriate level for later reference. Some specialists feel that giving AEDs in smaller, more frequent doses throughout the day may be preferable prior to a pregnancy.

Most women with epilepsy can expect a normal pregnancy and a normal healthy baby. However, there is an increased risk of complications and foetal malformations. The incidence of malformation in the general population is approximately 3 per cent, whereas in women with epilepsy the statistics indicate an increased incidence of approximately 4 per cent where severe abnormalities are studied and up to 50 per cent when minor abnormalities are included. The increase seems to depend on the dose and number of different drugs being taken (e.g. a woman on a small dose of one type of medication may have a smaller increased risk than a woman on higher doses or poly-therapy).

It is important to discuss at this stage the need for monitoring foetal abnormality with alpha-fetoproteins. The prospective parents may wish to discuss their feelings about the possible outcome and any action they would wish to take. It should be explained that they would be able to request a termination if an abnormality was identified. Some couples may decide not to undertake these procedures if they are not prepared to terminate a pregnancy.

Most major foetal abnormalities occur during the first 7–21 days following conception. Other problems such as cerebral migrational disorders may occur later in the first trimester. The risk of rebound seizures following the sudden withdrawal of medication also carries its own problems.

It is important to remember that tonic–clonic seizures can result in an increased risk of spontaneous abortion in early pregnancy. They may also lead to foetal cerebral damage due to hypoxia if multiple seizures occur during the pregnancy. Uncontrolled epilepsy also carries a risk of injury for the mother, and may cause continuing problems following the delivery.

The discontinuation or change of medication may also have social implications. If the woman has been seizure-free and is driving, she should be advised that she should not drive during and for 6 months after the withdrawal of her medication. This is not law, but it is a strong recommendation.

Some specific statistics

Research indicates that the approximate incidence of foetal abnormalities reported is:

- Approximately 2.5 per cent of babies born to mothers without epilepsy.
- Approximately 4.2 per cent of babies born to mothers with epilepsy and not on medication.
- Approximately 6 per cent of babies born to mothers with epilepsy and on medication (this figure will vary depending on the number of drugs and doses of drug being taken).

Not all of these abnormalities will be serious or life threatening.

Problems associated with the epilepsy

There is evidence that there is an increased risk of the following, possibly related to maternal seizures during the pregnancy:

- Ante-partum haemorrhage
- Spontaneous abortion
- Premature rupture of the membranes
- Premature birth
- Low birth weight
- Neonatal death.

Problems associated with the drugs

1. *Phenytoin*:
   - cleft lip and palate
   - dysmorphic features
   - craniofacial abnormalities
   - foetal phenytoin syndrome.
2. *Sodium valproate*:
   - neural tube defect (higher at doses of more than 1000 mg/day – 1–2 per cent risk)
   - foetal valproate syndrome (dysmorphic features and developmental delay)
   - cardiovascular abnormality
   - urogenital malformations
   - developmental delay.
3. *Carbamazepine*:
   - neural tube defect (0.9 per cent)
   - reduced head circumference
   - dysmorphic features.

Developmental delay was thought to be a problem with carbamazepine, although recent research does not support this.

At present there is insufficient evidence to say whether lamotrigine, gabapentin and tiagabine carry any risks. Vigabatrin and topiramate have produced abnormalities in animal studies.

The pregnancy

> Epilepsy was recently reported to be the second largest cause of maternal death in the UK, but many maternity units have no specific policy for dealing with epilepsy and pregnancy as they would for diabetes and pregnancy!

Antenatal care should follow normal local practice. If there is a local epilepsy specialist nurse or a midwife with a specific interest in epilepsy, the woman should be in contact with him or her. Try to establish what your local service can provide and whether there is a formal referral system.

Women with epilepsy should be monitored during the pregnancy by the community midwife in the same way as any other women; however, they should also be under the care of an obstetrician. They should be able to have a vaginal delivery and the same choice of pain control available to other women. Any intervention should be on obstetric grounds.

There is now a national register in the UK to collect information about pregnancy outcomes. Women who become pregnant can register themselves by calling the free telephone number 0800 389 1248.

The first trimester

The main problems at this stage of the pregnancy will be associated with possible nausea and vomiting, which may result in the woman being unable to take the medication. If this becomes a problem, medical advice should be sought before it can affect seizure control. Contact should be established with a local service to enable monitoring of both the epilepsy and the pregnancy. Drug levels may need to be checked.

The second trimester

In this trimester the women should be monitored as necessary, with alpha-fetoproteins measured and a high-density scan undertaken to monitor growth and possible foetal abnormalities. Counselling should be available if any abnormalities are found. It will be important to try and establish whether or not any abnormality is related to the anti-epileptic medication. This will have psychological implications for the couple.

The epilepsy control should be monitored and drug levels checked if appropriate. If any change in medication is to be made, this should be undertaken by the specialist responsible for the epilepsy care.

The third trimester

In this trimester it is important to monitor the seizure control and to check drug levels if appropriate. The drugs may need to be adjusted, as at this stage the increase in body weight and blood volume may result in dilution of the serum concentration. Potential problems at the delivery should be discussed before the birth plan is established, so that avoiding actions can be written into it. These may include potential triggers and pain relief during the delivery.

1. *Potential triggers.* Some of these may not have an effect at the time of delivery, but may have an impact following the delivery:
   * stress and anxiety
   * lack of sleep, exhaustion due to prolonged labour
   * missing medication
   * hyperventilation.
2. *Pain relief during the delivery.* Women with epilepsy should have access to all normally used methods of pain relief. However, they should be informed of potential problems so that they can make an informed choice about the methods used. The following should be considered:
   * Entonox is safe if used properly, although hyperventilation during use should be avoided
   * TENS machines are considered safe, but some women find these ineffective
   * An epidural anaesthetic is considered the safest option, although the anaesthetist should be informed of the diagnosis of epilepsy
   * Birthing pools are not often recommended because of the small risk of a seizure while in the pool
   * Pethidine can cause vomiting, which will affect the retention of other medication. While there has been some anecdotal reports of increased incidence of seizures associated with the use of pethidene during delivery, there is no definite evidence at present; although the BNF states that this

drug should be used with caution in people with convulsive disorders.

All women on liver enzyme-inducing anticonvulsant drugs (carbamazepine, phenytoin, barbiturates, and probably topiramate) should be prescribed vitamin K (phytomenadione) 20 mg daily for the last 4 weeks of the pregnancy. This is because of the increased incidence of haemorrhagic disease of the newborn. The baby should also be given vitamin K according to local protocol.

The delivery

Most women with epilepsy will have a normal vaginal delivery. If this is not possible, it is usually because of an obstetric reason and not because of the epilepsy. Women with epilepsy are at high risk of problems during the delivery, and because of this it is advisable that deliveries are undertaken in a unit that can provide any necessary intervention for both mother and baby. Consideration should be given to potential triggers for seizures before the birth plan is written. This will not only help to reduce the risk of seizures during the delivery but will also help the women to feel empowered about any actions that are taken. Approximately 1–2 per cent of women with epilepsy have a seizure at the time of delivery. Care needs to be taken, as the delivery may progress uneventfully although there will still be an increased risk of seizures for some days following the delivery.

Childcare and safety

Breast-feeding: this is recommended if the woman wishes to breastfeed. The baby will have been exposed to the drug from conception, and the levels in the breast milk will be less than those passing via the placenta during the pregnancy. However, if the baby is very drowsy or excessively irritable this may need to be reconsidered.

Bathing, feeding and carrying: advice should be given about precautions when undertaking these tasks shortly after the delivery. Even if the woman has been seizure-free and the delivery has gone well, there may still be a slightly increased risk of a seizure during the post-partum period because of the trigger factors for seizures during the delivery.

- Bathing the baby may be safer if undertaken when a member of the family can be present. If this is not possible the baby should be washed on a safe surface, with a small bowl of water placed away from the baby, and not put into the bath.
- Feeding and nursing should be done in as safe an environment as possible – if necessary, on a large chair or on the floor surrounded by cushions.
- It may be better to avoid carrying the baby, especially on stairs. Consideration may need to be given to using a buggy to take the baby from room to room, or strapping the baby into a carrycot while negotiating stairs.
- The mother should try to avoid becoming overtired. Even if she wishes to breastfeed, it may be possible to express the milk into a bottle so that she does not have to give every feed. (She will probably still wake but can stay in bed.)

General safety

Special consideration may be needed for women with uncontrolled epilepsy in the form of help with childcare so they can maintain their independence. Items such as safety brakes for prams and pushchairs are available, and provision may need to be made for the mother to attend a mother and baby group as soon as possible. Extra visits from the midwife and health visitor may also help if the family is having difficulty coping. The local epilepsy specialist nurse, if available, should be informed of the delivery and any problems; he or she may be able to help.

Epilepsy was recently reported as the second largest cause of maternal death in the UK. We need to improve services!
- Women with epilepsy should be referred for specialist advice about epilepsy and pregnancy
- Women with epilepsy should be reassured that most will have a normal pregnancy with a normal vaginal delivery
- Pregnancies should be planned and folic acid 5 mg daily taken for at least 3 months prior to the pregnancy and for

the first 3 months of the pregnancy; some units advise continuing the folic acid throughout the pregnancy
- If the pregnancy is not planned, any radical change in medication on discovery of a pregnancy is not advisable
- Women should have their epilepsy closely monitored during pregnancy
- Some women may need their medication adjusting to prevent loss of seizure control during pregnancy
- Women with epilepsy should have access to alpha-feto-protein screening and high-resolution detailed scans during their pregnancy
- Women with epilepsy should have skilled counselling ane support during the screening process
- Oral Vitamin K 20 mg daily should be given to the mother for the last 4 weeks of the pregnancy if she is taking carbamazepine, phenytoin, topiramate, primidone or any of the barbiturates; this helps to reduce the risk of haemorrhagic disease of the newborn
- Advice should be given about safety related to caring for the baby
- The mother should be reminded about possible problems with contraception, depending on her medication; this could have been the reason for this pregnancy if it was unplanned.

EPILEPSY AND THE MENOPAUSE

There is very little information available regarding the effects of the menopause on epilepsy and seizure control; very few studies have been undertaken, and those that have were flawed and therefore not helpful.

There is an increased risk of osteoporosis in both sexes if there has been long-term use of phenytoin, primidone or carbamazepine, as these are known to accelerate the metabolism of vitamin D and therefore increase the risk of this condition. Hormone replacement therapy is recommended for women with epilepsy. This should follow the same criteria as for any other women, and should be a combination of oestrogen and progestogen. This is because of the reported increased incidence of seizures in women given oestrogen-only treatment. The method of administration does not appear to be relevant. There are no recommendations regarding the doses to be used, although if no benefit is felt when treatment is introduced it may be that the dose needs to be increased. Vitamin D and calcium supplements may also need to be considered.

11 Epilepsy in the elderly

INTRODUCTION

Do we need to consider epilepsy in the elderly as being any different to that in the adult population? There is now much evidence that there are different presentations of symptoms to be considered, and that the social impact on this age group is different than on other adults. The elderly may not be able to cope as well, and greater support may be needed.

INCIDENCE AND PREVALENCE

The incidence and prevalence of epilepsy in the elderly have changed over recent decades as life expectancy has increased and more people have survived to live with cerebrovascular damage. Approximately 30 per cent of all newly diagnosed cases of epilepsy each year are in people over the age of 65 years. The prevalence of treated epilepsy in people over the age of 70 years is now thought to be double that in children. The most common cause of epilepsy in the elderly is cerebrovascular disease and, as there has been an increase in this condition over the last five decades, this is almost certainly the reason for the change in statistics. Approximately 0.7 per cent of the elderly population are now treated for epilepsy, and it is the third most common neurological condition in this age group after dementia and stroke.

THE IMPLICATIONS OF LATE ONSET EPILEPSY

The onset of epilepsy at any age will carry many lifestyle implications, and some may consider that if its onset occurs after a person's working life has naturally ended then some of its impact will be lessened. However, a diagnosis of epilepsy can be as devastating in the elderly as in any age group:

- It may be that they grew up in a generation when epilepsy was not talked about and many myths existed, and they may believe it to be a mental health problem
- They may be afraid to talk about their symptoms if they have been experiencing 'weird' symptoms, as can occur with partial seizures
- The onset of seizures may lead to a loss of independence, with the family becoming more overprotective or the person no longer being confident to be left alone or to undertake such tasks as shopping or visiting friends without an escort
- Elderly people may be more dependent on motorized transport and find using public transport difficult; the loss of their driving licence will add to restrictions on their lifestyle, and there is less likelihood of it being returned even if they become seizure-free
- Individual seizures may result in greater morbidity in older people than in younger people as the elderly are at greater risk of fractures and loss of confidence – they may fear that they will die in a seizure.

DIAGNOSIS

Making a diagnosis of epilepsy in the elderly can be as difficult as making a correct diagnosis in children. There are many factors that may confuse the history and lead to an incorrect diagnosis:

- Seizures may not be as stereotyped and may present in an unexpected manner
- It may be more difficult to obtain a history or eyewitness accounts if the person lives alone
- Many of the symptoms described may be due to other causes common in the elderly
- Co-existing cognitive failure in the patient and the spouse may make the history less reliable.

Differential diagnosis

Alternative causes of loss of consciousness, falls or confusional states to be considered in the age group include:

- Syncope – causes may be cardiac, blood pressure changes or postural
- Hypoglycaemia
- Transient ischaemic attacks
- Transient global amnesia
- Vertigo
- Non-specific dizziness, which can affect up to 10 per cent of this age group.

Seizures may present as:

- Acute confusional state
- Fluctuating mental or cognitive function
- Repeated falls or injury.

They may be misdiagnosed as:

- Increased clumsiness
- Psychiatric disorders
- Dementia
- Cerebrovascular disease
- Functional problems.

The diagnosis can be particularly difficult if the person lives alone or has recently lost a partner, and if co-morbidity with one of these problems exists.

Epilepsy in relation to other conditions

Cerebrovascular disease

Cerebrovascular disease (CVD) accounts for between 30 and 50 per cent of all cases of epilepsy in the elderly. There may not always be an established diagnosis of cerebrovascular disease prior to the onset of the seizures; this may only become apparent when an episode of loss of consciousness or confusion is being investigated. Seizures may not always present at the time of a recognized episode of stroke. This can be a problem for both the person and the family, as they may still be trying to come to terms with one condition that has changed their lives when a second problem is brought to their attention. Even though medically the two problems are related it is often difficult for the person and family to accept this, particularly if there has been a time lapse between their presentations.

- Evidence of a past episode of CVD, previously undiagnosed, will be found on investigation in approximately 15 per cent of elderly patients with late onset epilepsy and no obvious underlying cause
- At the time of a stroke, approximately 5 per cent of patients will develop seizures
- Within 5 years of a stroke, approximately 10 per cent of patients will develop seizures.

The incidence of seizures seems higher in haemorrhagic stroke rather than in ischaemic stroke.

Some causes of cerebrovascular disease in the elderly that would need to be excluded are:

- Rheumatic heart disease
- Endocarditis
- Valvular (heart) disease
- Cardiac dysrhythmias.

Additional underlying causes of epilepsy

- Cerebral tumours (usually metastatic or gliomas) are present in between 5 and 15 per cent of elderly patients presenting with late onset epilepsy
- Metabolic conditions e.g. alcohol, dehydration, pyrexia, renal or hepatic problems, infection
- Subdural haematoma
- Cerebral aneurysm
- Drugs (many prescribed drugs are epileptogenic, and the elderly are more likely to be on medication).

INVESTIGATING EPILEPSY IN THE ELDERLY

Neuroimaging should be undertaken to exclude tumours and to establish any evidence of cerebrovascular disease. If there is an established diagnosis of CVD, imaging will help to establish any recent extension of the condition.

The use of EEG in the care of epilepsy has previously been discussed. It is not necessarily a diagnostic tool because of the variants that may exist within a normal record, and this becomes even more problematic in the elderly:

- There may be increased slow wave activity in the temporal lobe, particularly on the left
- Small sharp spikes may occur during drowsing or sleep
- There may be runs of temporoparietal activity
- Cerebrovascular disease may produce focal and bilateral temporal lobe changes that are not epilepsy.

TREATMENT OF EPILEPSY IN THE ELDERLY

Little research information is available regarding drug treatment in the elderly. Drug trials often exclude the older patients. Decisions about drug treatment are often made on the basis of recommended adult regimens without consideration of additional factors.

When deciding the most appropriate treatment, the individual's needs and any potential problems should be considered. The elderly already have an increased risk of conditions such as osteoporosis, and may have reduced renal or hepatic function, which will influence the choice of treatment initiated. Other factors to be considered include the decreased metabolic rate of the elderly and possible memory impairment.

The above factors can result in altered pharmacokinetics, leading to increased serum levels and an extended half-life of drugs, and also problems with compliance. In addition, the reduced cerebral reserve can result in an increased incidence of side effects at 'therapeutic' serum levels.

Medication

When choosing medication, the following factors should be considered for each individual:

- Age
- Level of family support
- Underlying cause of the epilepsy
- Additional medical problems
- Medication for other conditions.

When introducing medication:

- Commence at the lowest possible dose
- Increase the dose slowly
- Try to achieve control at the lowest possible dose
- Try to achieve control on monotherapy
- Monitor the patient at regular, frequent intervals to aid compliance
- Establish telephone contact if possible
- Provide support and explanation to the patient, carer and family to help promote understanding and confidence.

Some potential problems

- Liver enzyme-inducing drugs, including phenytoin and carbamazepine, carry an increased risk of osteoporosis, hypertension and cardiac dysrhythmias
- The risk of drug interaction is greater because of the increased incidence of many other medical problems resulting in the person being on polytherapy for multiple conditions.

Drug interactions are discussed in Chapter 7.

12 Epilepsy in the learning disabled

INTRODUCTION

Looking after people with learning difficulties is hard at the best of times, but when the matter at issue is epilepsy, with its diagnosis dependent on clinical observation and its drug treatments associated with cognitive impairment, care of this patient group tests the skills of the best health care professionals. However, when it is successful the management of patients with learning disability can be very rewarding.

INCIDENCE OF EPILEPSY IN PEOPLE WHO HAVE A LEARNING DISABILITY

The incidence of epilepsy in people with learning disability will vary depending on the degree of disability and the underlying problem that has resulted in the disability presenting. On average, 30 per cent of people with a mild to moderate learning disability and 50 per cent of people with a severe learning disability are affected.

Some specific incidences include:

- Down's syndrome   2%
- Fragile X syndrome   10–25%
- Rett's syndrome   70–80%
- Tuberous sclerosis   80%
- Sturge–Weber syndrome   80%

MAKING THE DIAGNOSIS

This should be undertaken following the same recommendations as for any other group. Other causes of seizures will need to be considered. This group can present with non-epileptic attack disorder, or the problem may be behavioural. Investigations will need to be undertaken, although the individual's ability to cope and understand should be taken into consideration. The fact that people have a learning disability should not exclude them from services available to others.

Seizure presentation

Seizure presentation may vary in people with learning disabilities because of the altered function of the brain resulting from the underlying structural changes. This will make the recognition of specific seizure types more difficult, and therefore complicate the process of diagnosis.

Communication

Communication with people with moderate or severe learning difficulties is likely to be problematic or impossible. It may be limited to non-verbal communication, with carers or health care professionals trying to communicate on the individual's behalf – acting as an advocate, with the person's best interests at heart. People with a learning disability will have relatives and/or a key worker with whom communication is particularly important, as the usual channels will not be open. Key workers are able to provide invaluable information about the phenomenology of attacks, their frequency, and associated behavioural changes. They are fundamental in instituting any change in therapeutic regimen and monitoring for side effects. Their input will be invaluable when trying to distinguish possible seizures from behavioural problems.

ANTI-EPILEPTIC DRUG TREATMENT

Prescribing for people with learning disabilities is often a more difficult process than in the non-disabled population. They are prone to associated complications that may result in compromised cognitive function, communication difficulties and atypical seizure types. They may also be on concomitant medication. The main problem will be establishing the effectiveness of the medication and any side effects, due to the person's lack of effective communication skills.

Initiating medication

It is good practice with any patient to start at a low dose and titrate the drug slowly, allowing an adequate period of time between dose changes to monitor the effect of the medication. It is essential to monitor behavioural changes closely for both positive and negative effects. Serum blood levels are rarely necessary, except in the monitoring of phenytoin. Serum blood monitoring of other drugs often leads to unnecessary increases or reductions in dosage, which subsequently affect seizure control. Occasionally monitoring may be required if the patient lacks the verbal skills to communicate side effects and subsequent inadvertent intoxication may occur.

As the therapeutic window for anti-epileptic drugs is very narrow, skilled observation by well-informed carers is often the key to determining whether intoxication is present. Depending on the level of additional disability, the normally recognized symptoms of diplopia and ataxia may not be appropriate markers. It may be that increased drowsiness and altered behaviour are more commonly seen symptoms. Irritability or rubbing of the eyes or head may be signs that a person is experiencing unpleasant symptoms although he or she cannot communicate this in any other way. The person may become clumsier or develop difficulties in feeding because of co-ordination. Monitoring serum anticonvulsant levels may not be an appropriate way of establishing problems. It is also possible to have symptoms of toxicity with levels that are reported to be within the therapeutic range where carbamazepine and lamictal are used in conjunction, and some individuals are more sensitive to particular medication and may develop symptoms of toxicity on low doses.

Whilst monitoring behaviour, the changes may be negative (e.g. irritability, aggressiveness) or positive (e.g. awakening, increased alertness). It is important to remember that positive changes may be misinterpreted, and thus the client who 'wakes up' and becomes somewhat more demanding of carers may be seen as behaviourally disturbed as they may not be as compliant with social behaviour or tasks as in the past. These changes may in fact be due to improved seizure control leading to the person being more active and beginning to establish his or her own personality.

Drugs used in the treatment of people with a learning disability

All anti-epileptic drugs should be used with caution in the learning disabled.

Vigabatrin is now rarely used because of the problem of visual field defects; it has still been included in the drug information for reference, as it is occasionally used in very specific situations.

The following is basic information; as with any other group of patients, the drugs and doses used need to be tailored to the individual.

Preferred drugs include carbamazepine, gabapentin, lamotragine and sodium valproate, because they are broad-spectrum drugs and may have a lower side effect profile.

Drugs to be used with caution include phenytoin, phenobarbitone, topiramate and vigabatrin, because there is a higher risk of side effects. These drugs are only used in specific situations.

Accurate record keeping is essential from the family and carers in order to establish the effectiveness and side effects of the medication.

BEHAVIOURAL PROBLEMS AND EPILEPSY

Distinguishing between behavioural disturbance and epileptic activity can be very difficult in people with learning disability due to the complexity of their epilepsy and/or their behaviour pattern in general. When assessing a situation, care should always be taken to ensure that additional physical health problems have been considered. Challenging behaviour in people with epilepsy may be categorized as follows:

1. Challenging behaviour caused by seizures. This is challenging behaviour that is present before, during, and after the seizure, does not occur at any other time, and is linked directly to the seizure activity of the individual.
2. Challenging behaviour caused by anti-epileptic medication.
3. Behavioural problems independent of seizures or medications. This is when challenging behaviour occurs independently of the seizures and is not related to the dose of the medication.

Challenging behaviour caused by seizures

Some epileptic seizures can present as challenging behaviour. Things to look for in aiding distinction are:

- Is there stereotyped behaviour that occurs prior to a definable seizure?
- Does the behaviour occur independently of any external factors known to cause problems with behaviour?
- Is the observed behaviour the same each time that it occurs – e.g. same body movements, facial expression, or vocalization?
- Is the person confused or drowsy after the behaviour problem?

All behavioural problems need to be recorded accurately at the time by an observer.

Challenging behaviour caused by medication

The following anti-epileptic medication can cause behavioural problems:

- Phenobarbitone, particularly in children
- Sodium valproate, which may cause increased agitation, aggression, and hyperactivity
- Vigabatrin, may cause problems in 5 per cent of patients
- Topiramate, which can cause depression.

Some medication, such as carbamazepine, is known to have a stabilizing effect on mood changes. The withdrawal of this type of anti-epileptic drug and its antipsychotic action may well see the emergence or subsequent return of psychiatric symptomatology or behavioural disturbance, if the drug that is withdrawn was previously suppressing them.

Behavioural problems independent of seizures or medication

In most cases the behavioural problem will not be related in any way to the seizures or the medication.

Differentiating behavioural problems

- Does the challenging behaviour observed/identified always occur before or after specific incidents?
- Is the behaviour related to specific people, activities, places, times or environments?
- Is the behaviour controlled or changed by direct intervention?

Who can help with behavioural problems?

Locally there may be community learning disability health teams (CLDHT) who can help with these problems. These often consist of community nurses, specialist nurses, psychologists, occupational therapists, speech therapists, sensory nurses and consultant psychiatrists. Members of the team may be able to offer help and support, but should aim to work closely with the neurologist or learning disability consultant providing the care for the person's epilepsy.

SUMMARY

In learning disabled people with epilepsy:

- The diagnosis of epilepsy may be difficult to establish
- Drug treatment will be more difficult to monitor

- Behavioural difficulties are common, but are not always associated with seizures
- Non-epileptic seizures may develop
- Good communication between professionals is essential to providing good care.

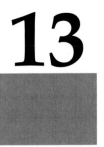

13

Clinical audit and data collection associated with epilepsy care and services

INTRODUCTION

Data collection has always been a part of nursing practice, as activities in relation to direct patient care are documented. This is usually an ongoing practice not specifically undertaken in relation to an audit project. Clinical audit is now also a well-established part of nursing practice, relying on data collection in relation to a specific project that will culminate in a report of the data collected. In this chapter we will discuss ways in which these activities can be applied to epilepsy care.

> Clinical audit is the critical examination of patient care in order to identify any shortcomings, the introduction of change designed to remedy the shortcomings, and the subsequent re-audit of the case to determine if improvements have occurred.

ONGOING DATA COLLECTION

Data collection may be introduced as an ongoing means of logging workload activity and patient contact. If collected in a consistent format, this information may also become the basis of a local audit. Amassing the information on a computer in a Microsoft Access program may be the better option for analyses; Microsoft Excel is adequate for some uses but may restrict the method of analysis available.

TYPES OF CLINICAL AUDIT

A clinical audit can be as large as the national audit commissioned by the government in 1996 and undertaken by the Clinical Standards Advisory Group. The research for the audit commenced in November 1997, and the report was produced in June 1999 (Clinical Standards Advisory Group, 1999). Other recent national audits in epilepsy include a survey of the experience and attitudes of people with epilepsy (British Epilepsy Association, 2000) and a national audit of service by the Epilepsy Task Force (1998). Audits may also be undertaken within specific units (such as Neuroscience units) or within a NHS trust or primary care group (e.g. Mills *et al.*, 1999), or may involve one nurse auditing his or her own activity. Audit may be on general aspects of patient care or satisfaction, or may be more specific – e.g. on epilepsy and pregnancy services.

Ongoing national audits include:

- The UK Epilepsy and Pregnancy Register, co-ordinated by Dr J. Morrow, Consultant Neurologist, Department of Neurology (Ward 21), Royal Victoria Hospital, Grosvenor Road, Belfast, BT12 6BA (Telephone 01232 240503, Ext. 4325; Freephone 01232 235258).
- The National Sentinel Audit Project – an audit of epilepsy-related deaths at national level. Deaths need to be reported to Epilepsy Bereaved by the family of the deceased. The relevant data will then be collected.

UNDERTAKING AUDIT

For many people, audit is a task in which they will be involved but they will not initiate. Audit does not need to be complex; on occasions more information can be gained from a simple audit that can be easily analysed than from a more complicated audit. Some of the following ideas can be adapted for use by any nurse involved in epilepsy care at whatever level. Others may be more appropriate in particular clinical settings.

Undertaking local audit

This can be done in primary care at trust (group) or practice level. In secondary care it could be undertaken within a specific unit – neurology, paediatrics, learning disability, obstetrics or accident and emergency. In both primary and secondary care there will usually be a clinical audit department or a source of help with this activity.

If you are interested in undertaking audit in any aspect of epilepsy care you should first discuss this with your manager or head of department, as audit can be time consuming. Have a basic outline of the audit you would like to undertake, and if possible try to be specific.

When considering undertaking an audit, you will need to know:

- What information you want to audit
- Where you will collect the information
- Whether this will involve patient or staff questioners
- How you will record the data
- How the data will be analysed
- How the outcome will be used
- How the audit will help patient care.

Establishing contact with your local clinical audit department and asking for their assistance may help. There may be a clinical nurse specialist in epilepsy locally who could help. If audit is to be related to improving patient care, you will need to find standards by which your results can be judged; others may already have undertaken similar audit.

For specialist nurses interested in auditing their workload and activity, it may help to be able to compare outcomes with other specialist nurse activity.

Data collected can be logged as different categories:

- Patient data
- Nurse workload data
- Patient knowledge
- Outcomes of training sessions held.

Many audits would not include all the data listed below, but would concentrate on specific sections depending on your audit criteria and outcome needs. A more general audit giving basic information may be a better starting point, leading to further audit in the future.

Information suitable for audit

- Identifying patient caseload
- Age range and sex of patients
- Age at onset of epilepsy
- Frequency and type of review – primary/secondary care, medical/nursing
- Co-morbidity
- Drug review – number of drugs per patient, dose ranges, side effects, any changes made and reasons for change
- Compliance problems
- Advice given
- Source of referral
- Follow-up or discharge
- Referrals to other services, type of referral and reasons
- Assessing standard of documentation
- Patient satisfaction.

Basic primary care audit

A basic primary care audit may be used as a starting point to identify the caseload of patients with epilepsy within a practice, and essential information to look at current practice. This type of audit would need to be undertaken with the agreement of practice staff with a timescale for completion included. A report should be compiled and the results presented at a practice meeting, which would allow discussion on outcomes and future actions. This audit would also act as a basis for a practice disease register if one did not already exist.

Outcome agreements may be:

- To continue updating the register
- To arrange review of patients not seen within an agreed timescale.

Identifying patients in primary care

Patients in primary care can be identified by:

1. Undertaking a search for repeat prescriptions, although this method will not necessarily be accurate for the following reasons:
   - newly diagnosed patients may not be receiving repeat prescriptions
   - patients may be undergoing drug changes and not receiving repeat prescriptions
   - prescriptions may have been issued at the surgery or on home visits
   - patients may not be compliant and therefore not collecting their prescriptions
   - patients may have had their medication stopped although their diagnosis still stands
   - some anti-epileptic drugs are also used to treat neuropathic pain (e.g. carbamazepine, gabapentin, lamotrigine)
   - some anti-epileptic drugs are used in the treatment of some psychiatric conditions, e.g. carbamazepine.
2. Using the practice disease register, if there is one.
3. Identifying the patients on anti-epileptic medication and then reviewing their notes to establish the diagnosis.

The more methods you have to capture patients, the more complete but time-consuming your audit will be.

Secondary care audit

The way this is undertaken will depend on the area of care in which the audit is to be undertaken and the potential patient throughput to be audited. It may be that a timescale for identifying patients will need to be set. The hospital information system may or may not provide a useful tool for identifying patients, and an audit of all patients attending may be necessary to identify the patients seen with epilepsy.

For example, consider the following points:

- Set a timescale for identifying patients
- Choose specific clinics or a unit to be audited
- Identify staff to undertake the audit
- Design audit sheets for recording the information depending on agreed outcomes

• Identify a method of data analysis.

Auditing nurse work activity relating to epilepsy

Auditing activity does not have to be reserved for specialist nurses; it may be that this could be undertaken by a practice or school nurse, or by midwives in an obstetric unit. Work analysis could be recorded on a weekly basis. Within this type of audit you may wish to include:

• Number of patients seen
• Number of telephone contacts
• Meetings attended
• Teaching sessions held
• Training sessions attended
• Hours worked
• Annual leave taken.

SAMPLE AUDIT SHEETS

Tables 13.1 and 13.2 are basic ideas for use in auditing epilepsy care and services. They will need to be adjusted to meet individual needs, or you will need to develop your own audit tool to record data to meet the needs of the audit criteria set. The data collection sheet may become very large if all drugs are included, so it may be wise to have an appendix sheet of drugs with a code to be used in the original sheet.

If you wish to present the information you will need to ensure that each patient is allocated an identification (ID) number as well as personal details.

DATA PROTECTION

Clinical audits contain confidential information about patients. This may or may not be easily linked back to the individual person. As health care professionals we have a duty of confidentiality and have to safeguard any databases we have responsibility for. If you are in doubt regarding what you can do with a database, or have worries about confidentiality, the data protection officer of your institution should be able to give specific guidance.

Table 13.1 Sample audit sheet to identify patient caseload and standard of documentation

Patient	1	2	3	4	5
ID number					
Name					
DOB					
Sex					
Age of onset of epilepsy					
Seen by neurologist Y/N/not recorded (NR)					
Number of drugs for epilepsy					
Names of drugs for epilepsy					
Last review primary care (PC) for epilepsy					
Last review PC not for epilepsy					
Last review secondary care (SC) for epilepsy date/(NR)					
Seizures frequency recorded, number/(NR)					
Advice recorded on Contraception, date/(NR)					
Advice recorded on pregnancy, date/(NR)					
Advice recorded on driving, date/(NR)					
Advice recorded on education date/(NR)/not applicable (NA)					
Advice on employment date/ (NR)/(NA)					

Table 13.2 Audit of epilepsy and pregnancy to assess standard of care

Variable	1	2	3	4	5
Patient ID number					
Date of referral					
Name					
Hospital number					
Consultant					
Date of birth					
Folic acid					
Vitamin K					
Gestation at referral					
Estimated date of delivery					
Actual date of delivery					
Type of delivery					
Active epilepsy					
Seizure during labour					
Live birth					
Multiple birth					
Foetal abnormality					
Still birth/foetal death					
Miscarriage					
Maternal death					
Sudden infant death					
Counselling					
Anti-epileptic drugs					
Area of residence					

AUDIT OR RESEARCH?

There is often a fine line between audit and research. If you are not sure about any project that you wish to undertake or are asked to be involved with, it is better to check before you start. There will be a local ethics committee in your hospital or trust, and there should be someone there who can advise you about the need for ethical approval for your project. If this is needed, advice may be obtained regarding how this should be requested. If you are undertaking a project with your local audit department they should know whether ethical approval will be needed, but you should always check.

SUMMARY OF UNDERTAKING CLINICAL AUDIT

Before undertaking a clinical audit, the following points must be considered:

- Why do you want to undertake an audit?
- What information do you want to audit?
- Where/how will you collect the information?
- Has a timescale been established for undertaking the audit?
- Who will collect the data?
- How will you record the data?
- Who will design the audit sheets?
- Will the audit involve patient or staff questioners?
- How will questionnaires be distributed and collected?
- How will the data be analysed?
- How will the outcome(s) be used?

As with most projects, ask a simple question and you might get a useful answer. Ask a complex question, and the data and complexity of the clinical situation will overwhelm you. Be modest in your aims and you will be likely to succeed.

Appendices

Appendix 1: The use of rectal diazepam

Problems have been identified in different areas of our health authority with the use of rectal diazepam. These problems included:

- Inappropriate prescribing when the drug was not necessary
- Inappropriate doses being prescribed
- No regular review of doses being prescribed
- Inconsistency of advice about when to administer
- Continued repeat prescription when no longer needed.

The clinical nurse specialist in epilepsy and the neuroscience directorate's pharmacist compiled the following guidelines. They were then adopted for use within primary care and by some private health care providers following approval by the hospital's Clinical Risk Management Board.

GUIDELINES FOR THE USE OF RECTAL DIAZEPAM IN THE TREATMENT OF PROLONGED OR RECURRENT SEIZURES IN PEOPLE WITH EPILEPSY

Compiled by Linda Baddeley and Ann Watson, North Staffordshire Hospital (NHS) Trust

Rationale

Rectal diazepam is used as emergency treatment in cases of prolonged or cluster seizures, with the aim of rapid cessation of seizure activity. This is not an appropriate method of treatment for all patients, but may be necessary in specific circumstances. Individual care plans for administration are an essential part of good practice to avoid inappropriate prescribing.

Aim

The aim of these guidelines is to assist the doctor in providing information that will ensure that carers, professional and non-professional, administer the drug correctly and appropriately. The information should always be used in conjunction with a prescription issued by a member of medical staff, and is not to be used as an aid to nurse prescribing.

Establishing the normal seizure pattern

An important factor to be established before agreement can be made on the administration of rectal diazepam is a written record of the person's normal seizure pattern and duration of seizure, i.e. tonic–clonic phase of a generalized seizure or the average length of a partial seizure. If this has not been agreed, then the criteria for the use of rectal diazepam in prolonged episodes cannot be established.

It should be noted that rectal diazepam should very rarely be needed in the treatment of prolonged partial seizures unless the patient is distressed by the seizures.

Criteria for the use of rectal diazepam

If agreement is reached between doctor, patient (where possible) and carer that there may ever be a need for the use of rectal diazepam, then guidelines regarding its use should be clearly defined and written instructions provided. These should include:

- The duration of an individual seizure before administration, with definite instructions about the seizure type and which pattern of the seizure is to be timed
- If a definite pattern of cluster seizures is recognized, then how many seizures in a given time should be observed before the drug is administered
- How to monitor the effectiveness of the drug
- What action to take if the seizures continue after a recommended time
- Concerns of the patient.

The following should also be defined:

- The identification of any carers who will be administering the drug
- Training needs of the identified carers in the administration of the drug
- An agreed method of recording the amount of drug given and the outcome
- Timing – this needs to be confirmed by looking at a clock, as the carer's perception of time may be distorted by events.

Suggested timings on the duration of the seizure

In generalized seizures the tonic–clonic phase should not be allowed to continue for more than 3 minutes, or 2 minutes longer than the person's normal pattern, before the drug is administered.

In partial seizures it should only be administered if attacks are frequent and distressing, or if the patient has a persistent partial seizure lasting more than 15 minutes.

Contraindications

- Respiratory depression
- Acute pulmonary insufficiency
- Severe hepatic impairment
- Previous adverse reaction to diazepam.

Dosage guidelines

Diazepam rectal solution is currently available as Stesolid (Dumex), Rectubes (CP Pharmaceuticals) and Diazepam Rectal Tubes (Lagap); however, their dosage recommendations differ.

When prescribing diazepam it is important to achieve effective plasma levels of diazepam early to achieve arrest of seizures, but clinical experience suggests that repeated doses of diazepam are often prescribed because of inadequate initial dosing resulting in subtherapeutic plasma concentrations.

CP Pharmaceuticals has recently changed dosing recommendations for rectal diazepam. These new recommendations are based on an effective concentration being at least 250 ng/ml

(Remy *et al.*, 1992), and possibly as high as 600 ng/ml (Benet *et al.*, 1996). Levels of diazepam below 150–200 ng/ml may be ineffective (Agurall *et al.*, 1975). Taken together with pharmacokinetic data, this suggests that a dose of 0.5 mg/kg is appropriate for both children and adults. CP Pharmaceuticals' dosage is therefore based on patient weight. A single dose is administered, and should not be repeated for at least 12 hours.

Although Dumex and Lagap largely agree with this guidance in respect of dosages in children, their recommendations with regard to adult doses differ to those of CP Pharmaceuticals. Dumex and Lagap are continuing with their recommendations of 10 mg (5 mg in elderly patients). Dumex specify that the dosage may be repeated after 5 minutes. This has led to confusion when referring to product literature for guidance.

There are several reasons why a single dose, as recommended by CP Pharmaceuticals, should be preferred. In generalized seizures it is important to obtain seizure control as quickly as possible to reduce the risk of neuronal damage and (particularly in children) to prevent the risk of temporal lobe anoxia, resulting in resistant seizures in later life. If dosing is by body weight the dose should not be repeated for 12 hours; this is because of the long half-life of the drug. The anticonvulsant effect is however much shorter, and will depend on the plasma concentration prior to redistribution. If an adequate dosage is ineffective, provided it has been administered correctly, this should identify the need to seek urgent hospital referral.

The current *British National Formulary* (*BNF*, 1998) recommends 500 mcg/kg (250 mcg/kg in the elderly) – i.e. largely in agreement with CP Pharmaceuticals' recommendation. However, recommendations that require knowledge of patient weight in kilograms can result in delayed administration, as this information is not always readily available.

The following guidelines have been designed in order to simplify administration.

A once-only dose of rectal diazepam should be used for the treatment of acute seizures, as in Table A1.1.

Side effects

Most common   Sedation, headaches, muscle weakness, dizziness, ataxia, confusion

Table A1.1 Rectal diazepam: proposed dose regime for acute treatment of seizures. The patient's weight should be used as a guide for the dose in preference to their age

Age	Weight	Rectal diazepam dose
< 1 year	< 10 kg	Not recommended
1–3 years	10–15 kg	5 mg
3–12 years	16–39 kg	10 mg
> 12 years	40–60 kg	15 mg
Adults	approx.< 60 kg or < 9 stones	20 mg
Adults	approx. > 60 kg or > 9 stones	30 mg
Elderly	Set dose. Use should be avoided where possible, especially in cases of renal/hepatic dysfunction 10 mg	

Rare	Dry mouth, jaundice, hypotension, bradycardia, chest pain, respiratory depression, apnoea

This list is not exhaustive; please refer to current *BNF* or manufacturer's information for further guidance.

Approval received from Clinical Risk Management and Director of Nursing Services, North Staffs Hospital Trust, 10 December 1998.

Review date: June 2002.

REFERENCES

Agurall, S., Berlin, A., Ferngren, H. *et al.* (1975). Plasma levels of diazepam after parenteral and rectal administration in children. *Epilepsia*, **16,** 227–83.

Benet, L. Z., Oie, S. and Schwartz, J. B. (1996). Design and optimisation of dosage regimens; pharmacokinetic data. In: *Goodman and Gilman's The Pharmacological basis of Therapeutics*, 9th edn (J.G. Hardman and L. E. Limbird, eds), pp. 1707–92. McGraw-Hill.

British National Formulary (1998). British Medical Association.

Remy, C., Jourdil, N., Villemain, D. *et al.* (1992). Intrarectal diazepam in epileptic adults. *Epilepsia*, **33(2),** 353–8.

CARE PROTOCOL FOR THE ADMINISTRATION OF RECTAL DIAZEPAM AS A FIRST AID MEASURE ONLY IN PEOPLE WITH EPILEPSY

Patient information

1. Name _____ Age _____

2. Address _____

3. GP _____Consultant _____

4. Type of seizure (include description) _____

_____

_____

5. Usual duration of the seizure _____

6. Additional information (possible trigger factors)

_____

_____

7. If this drug has been used before on this patient any known previous response or reaction

_____

_____

People trained to administer rectal diazepam to this person (to be completed by medical or nursing staff following training)

1. _____

2. _____

3. _____

TREATMENT PLAN FOR THE ADMINISTRATION OF RECTAL DIAZEPAM

1. Rectal diazepam should be given:
   a) If the tonic–clonic (shaking) part of a seizure has lasted longer than _____ minutes
   b) If a second seizure starts without full recovery from the first   yes/no
   c) If a partial seizure has lasted longer than 15 minutes and is distressing for the person having the seizure

   d) If there have been more than _____ partial seizures in a cluster (advice on this section should also depend on the distress being caused to the patient).

2. The dose of rectal diazepam to be given for this patient should be _____ mg as a single dose (see dosage chart in guidelines).

    _____

3. If there are any problems in administering the dose then please record action to be taken (e.g. ambulance called)

    _____

4. If there has been no response to the drug after 5 minutes call an ambulance.
    Ensure that ambulance staff and hospital staff are made aware of the dose of diazepam already given.

    _____

5. Always record the event, the amount of drug administered and the outcome including recovery time.

    _____

6. People to be notified at the time of an event

    _____

7. People to be notified of any event and its outcome

    _____

8. Telephone contact _____

Signature of prescribing physician _____

Review date of this advice _____

- Always try to carry out this procedure with as much privacy as possible for the person having the seizure
- Please remember that as you will be administering this drug while the person is having the seizure, so it may be a difficult procedure
- Where possible, two people should be present while this procedure is being undertaken.

Appendix 2: Information required by neurologist at out-patient appointment

PATIENT HISTORY

1. Please describe the patient's seizure/seizures in words.
Seizure type A

_____

(how many in last 12 months)

Seizure type B

_____

(how many in last 12 months)

2. How long has the patient been having seizures?

_____

3. Date of first seizure if occurred in the last 12 months.

_____

4. How often do the seizures occur?

Seizure type A Daily/weekly/monthly

Seizure type B Daily/weekly/monthly

5. Is there any history of febrile convulsions or seizures in the patient's infancy or childhood?

_____

6. Is there any family history of epilepsy or febrile convulsions?

_____

7. Please list all medication the patient is presently taking, including dosage and time.

_____

8. Does the patient have a diagnosed learning disability? Yes/No

9. If yes, does the patient have a diagnosed syndrome? Yes/No
   Please specify _____

10. Is the cause of the learning disability known, e.g.
    Birth trauma
    Infantile meningitis
    Head injury
    Other (please specify) _____

11. Does the patient have any other health problems at the present time?
    Yes/No   If Yes, please list

_____

_____

_____

Appendix 3: Patient information required by EEG department

Name _____

DOB _____

Has the patient had an EEG before? Yes/No
If yes, where was this carried out and what date?

_____

_____

When did the person last have an attack?

_____

Please describe in words how the patient's seizures/fits usually present themselves.

_____

_____

_____

_____

_____

Please list all medication the patient is taking at present.

_____

_____

_____

How co-operative is the patient usually?
       Very co-operative
       Can be unco-operative
       Very unco-operative

How co-operative is the patient in unfamiliar environments?

Very co-operative
Can be unco-operative
Very unco-operative

To provide the patient with adequate time and support to meet their needs, it is recommended that the patient is accompanied by someone who is familiar with him or her.

Appendix 4: Patient record card – sample 1

PATIENT DETAILS

Patient details: _____

Investigation: _____Date: _____
EEG _____
Ambulatory EEG_____
CT _____
MRI _____
Other _____

Diagnosis made by: Date of first seizure: _____
GP   Date of diagnosis: _____
Neurologist   Type of epilepsy: _____
Paediatrician   Type of seizure: _____
Other
Co-morbidity: Possible triggers:
1._____   1._____
2._____   2._____
3._____   3._____

Basic advice given:
Type/causes of epilepsy _____ Safety _____
Seizure types _____ Driving _____
First aid _____ Sources of information _____
Education _____
Employment _____
Contraception _____
Pregnancy _____

REVIEW INFORMATION

	1	2	3	4	5	6
Date of review						
Seizure frequency generalized per month						
Seizure frequency partial per month						
Seizure-free						
Date of last seizure						
AED 1						
AED 2						
AED 3						
New medication						
Drug discontinued						
Side effects						
Reason for change						
Compliance						
Additional medication						
Advice given Y/N						
Follow-up GP						
Follow-up specialist						

Appendix 5: Patient epilepsy information sheet – sample 2

The aim of this document is to improve patient monitoring and to help with future patient audit. Please complete in as much detail as possible when information is available.

Patient information label:

GP:
Consultant:
Referred to specialist nurse:
Yes / No

EPILEPSY PROFILE

Date of first seizure	Date of diagnosis	Epilepsy type	Seizure type

INVESTIGATION PROFILE

Investigation	First performed	Repeated	Comments
Standard EEG			
Sleep dep. EEG			
Ambulatory EEG			
CT scan			
MRI scan			

DRUG PROFILE

Drug	Date started	Date stopped + dose	Reason stopped

ADVICE GIVEN

Type	Date	Signature	Comment

Linda Baddeley CNS Epilepsy, revised January 2001.

Appendix 6: Information sheet for people newly diagnosed with epilepsy

MOST FREQUENTLY ASKED QUESTIONS

Q: Why me?

A: The doctor will probably not be able to answer this as in approximately 60 per cent of people with epilepsy no cause is found.

Q: What is epilepsy?

A: A disturbance in the electrical activity of the brain causing a seizure. It is sometimes thought of as an electrical storm in the brain.

Q: What is a seizure?

A: A sudden act of loss or altered consciousness resulting in involuntary movements or unusual sensations or thoughts.

Q: What were the tests for?

A: Sometimes *blood tests* are done to see if there are any medical problems that may have caused the seizure.

The *EEG* is to record the electrical activity of the brain to see if any irregularity is found that shows that you are at risk of having a seizure.

A *scan* is done to find whether there are any changes in the tissue of the brain that may be causing your seizures. This may be a CT scan, although where possible an MRI scan is better. Ask the doctor or nurse to explain the difference!

Q: What if an abnormality is found on the EEG?

A: This is electrical abnormality and if it fits with the diagnosis of epilepsy it may help confirm the diagnosis or tell the doctor the type of epilepsy. If it does not fit with the diagnosis of epilepsy, then the doctor will explain whether there is a problem. Not all changes are significant.

Q: What if there is an abnormality on the scan?

A: The doctor will explain this to you. Not all abnormalities are sinister; some may have been there from birth and have nothing to do with the epilepsy. The doctor will need to decide what treatment is needed, if any, and then explain it to you and arrange for this.

Q: **Could the doctor be wrong if all the test results are normal?**

A: It is not unusual for all the tests to be normal. This is one condition where the doctors need experience of working with people with epilepsy to be able to diagnose from the information they are given. They do sometimes get it wrong, particularly where the diagnosis is made too quickly.

Q: **How will I be treated?**

A: Usually with tablets to begin with, although other methods of treatment are available if necessary in the future.

Q: **Will the tablets stop the seizures?**

A: In about 70 per cent of people the seizures will be controlled when the tablets are started. If these do not work or they do not suit you, then the doctor can try other tablets. If the doctor thinks that other methods of treatment may help, he/she or the nurse will discuss these with you.

Q: **Is the doctor the only person who can help my family and me?**

A: In many areas there is a nurse who works specifically with people with epilepsy who the doctor can refer you to for further advice and support. Ask the doctor about this service.

Remember that if you have epilepsy you are entitled to free prescriptions. Ask for a P11 form at your chemist to apply.

OTHER FREQUENTLY ASKED QUESTIONS – ADDITIONAL INFORMATION THAT YOU MAY NEED

Q: **How does the diagnosis affect my ability to drive?**

A: You cannot drive on an ordinary licence until you have been seizure-free for 1 year. This applies even if you have only had one generalized seizure, or you have partial seizures with no loss of consciousness.

You can not hold an LGV or PCV licence until you have been seizure-free and off medication for 10 years.

For further advice about seizures that only occur at night, or driving if you are changing or stopping medication, you need to ask your specialist, GP or specialist nurse.

Q: **For children, will epilepsy or the medication affect their education?**

A: This will depend on the type of seizure and whether there are any side effects from the medication. You need to tell the teacher to ensure that the child receives appropriate help and does not miss lessons unnecessarily. The school nurse may be able to help to explain to the teachers.

Q: **Will the diagnosis of epilepsy or medication affect my employment?**

A: Usually not, but this will depend on the type of employment and the risk that having a seizure would cause to you or other employees. Your specialist or GP should be able to advise. If your employment will definitely be affected, if you discuss things with your employer they may be able to help.

Q: **If transport is a problem, can I get any help?**

A: Rail passes are available for people with epilepsy. New government guidelines now also mean that local bus passes are available if you have epilepsy. You need to check with your council offices; they do not necessarily mean free travel, but do allow concessions on fares.

Q: **Do the drugs affect the oral contraceptive or the contraceptive injection?**

A: Some drugs make the oral contraceptive less effective; you need to check with the doctor or specialist nurse. There is no evidence about the injection, although the advice is to be re-injected every 10 weeks.

Q: **Does having epilepsy or taking the medication affect my ability to have children?**

A: There are many issues associated with fertility and pregnancy, you should discuss these with your specialist or specialist nurse. Most women will be able to conceive, although you need to know the risk of the medication and the seizures on any pregnancy. You should take folic acid (a vitamin) 5 mg daily for at least 3 months prior to any pregnancy.

Q: **Am I entitled to other benefits?**

A: Having epilepsy entitles you to free prescriptions even if you remain in full-time employment. It does not necessarily entitle you to other benefits; you would need to enquire locally depending on your individual situation.

Q: **What about sport, leisure and other social activities?**

A: The advice will depend on your seizure type and how well controlled your epilepsy is. You need to discuss this with your doctor or specialist nurse. With correct advice and support, you should be able to continue most hobbies. You will need to consider how safe you would be if you had a seizure. Having epilepsy should not stop you from going on holiday. Changing your lifestyle unnecessarily will increase the impact of developing epilepsy; however, you do need to remember that you need to be sensible and safe. *Most people with epilepsy have a fulfilling and enjoyable life.*

Appendix 7: First aid during seizure

WHAT TO DO WHEN A MAJOR SEIZURE HAPPENS

- Do not attempt to move the person unless he or she is in danger. If necessary move any dangerous objects so that the person is not injured during the seizure.
- Place a soft object under the person's head to provide support, but ensure that it will not obstruct the airway.
- Do not try to restrain the person or put anything into the mouth.
- When the muscles have relaxed and the shaking has stopped, place the person onto his or her side in the recovery position.
- Wait with the person quietly and talk reassuringly. Some people may be a little confused after the attack, and this can be made worse by too much attention.
- Never try to give the person a drink until he or she asks for one. Swallowing may be affected until he or she is fully recovered.
- At an appropriate time it may be useful to describe what happens during the attack. This may help the person to feel less confused.
- Call an ambulance if the convulsive part of the seizure lasts for more than 3 minutes, if the person has a second seizure without fully recovering from the first, or if you are worried about his or her breathing.
- If to your knowledge this is the person's first seizure, then it may be better to get medical help.

WHAT SHOULD YOU DO IF A PARTIAL SEIZURE OCCURS?

Most partial seizures are short lasting with no danger of injury.

1. As with any seizure, get to know:
   - What will happen during the seizure
   - How long it will last
   - If the person has any warning that a seizure is about to occur
   - How the person feels and behaves after a seizure.
2. When one does occur:
   - Stay with the person
   - Talk to the person and provide reassurance
   - Remember that the person may be able to hear you even if he or she cannot answer
   - If the person starts to wander, do not try to use physical restraint as he or she may become difficult. Always try to use verbal commands unless the person is in real danger.
3. When the seizure is over:
   - Always record the event and how long it lasted
   - Ask the person what he or she remembers of the event
   - Make sure that the person doesn't have any gaps in remembering what was happening because of the seizure, as this may cause frustration later.

Appendix 8: Useful addresses

Useful addresses

Epilepsy Associations

British Epilepsy Association
Anstey House
40 Hanover Square
Leeds
Yorkshire LS3 1BE
Telephone 01132 2108800
Freephone helpline 0800 800 500

National Society for Epilepsy
Chalfont Centre for Epilepsy
Chalfont St Peter
Gerrards Cross
Buckingamshire SL8 0RJ
Telephone 01494 601300,
01494 601498 (outside office hours)
Helpline 01494 601400

Mersey Regional Epilepsy Association
The Glaxo Neurology Centre
Norton Street
Liverpool L3 8LR
Telephone 0151 2982666

Brainwave
The Irish Epilepsy Association
249 Crulin Road
Dublin 12
Telephone 003531 4557500

Gravesend Epilepsy Network
13 St George's Crescent
Gravesend
Kent DA12 4AR

Epilepsy Association of Scotland
48 Govan Road
Glasgow G51 1JL
Scotland
Telephone 0141427 4911

Enlighten, Action for Epilepsy
Edinburgh EH3 7AA
Scotland

Joint Epilepsy Council
PO Box 27027
Edinburgh
EH10 5YN
Telephone 0131 466 7155

Assessment centres

David Lewis Centre for Epilepsy
Mill Lane
Warford
Near Alderly Edge
Cheshire SK9 7UD
Telephone 01565 872613

National Hospital for Neurology and
Neurosurgery
Queen's Square
London WC1N 3BG
Telephone 0207 8373611

The Walton Centre for Neurology and
Neurosurgery
Rice Lane
Liverpool L9 1AE
Telephone 0151 5253611

Department of Neurology
Bootham Park Hospital
York YO3 7BY
Telephone 01904 454095

The Centre for Epilepsy
The Maudsley Hospital
De Crespigny Park
Camberwell
London SE5 8AZ
Telephone 0207 7036333

Chalfont Centre for Epilepsy
Chalfont St Peter
Gerrards Cross
Buckinghamshire SL8 0RJ
Telephone 01494 601300

Park Hospital for Children
Old Road
Headington
Oxford OX3 7LQ
Telephone 01865 741717

Department of Neuropsychiatry
Queen Elizabeth Psychiatric Hospital
Mindelsohn Way
Edgbaston
Birmingham B15 2TH
Telephone 0121 6782366

School for children with epilepsy

St Piers Lingfield Hospital School
St Piers Lane
Lingfield
Surrey RH7 6PW
Telephone 01342 832243

St Elizabeth's School
South End
Much Hadham
Hertfordshire SG10 6EW
Telephone 01279 843451

David Lewis Centre for Epilepsy
Mill Lane
Warford
Near Alderly Edge
Cheshire SK9 7UD
Telephone 01565 872613

Medical alert suppliers

Medic Alert Foundation
12 Bridge Wharf
156 Caledonian Road
London N1 9UU
Telephone 0207 833 3034

SOS Talisman
21 Gray's Court
Ley Street
Ilford
Essex IG2 7RQ

Tyser UK Ltd
Acorn House
Great Oakes
Basildon
Essex SS14 1AL
Telephone 01268 284361

Other useful addresses

For information on medical fitness to drive:
Drivers Medical Unit
DVLA, Swansea

For information on UK epilepsy and
pregnancy register:
Dr J Morrow
Consultant Neurologist
Department of Neurology (Ward 21)
Royal Victoria Hospital
Grosvenor Road
Belfast BT12 6BA
Telephone 01232 240503
Freephone helpline 0800 389 1248

Epilepsy Bereaved (a self help group for
family and friends of SUDEP victims):
PO Box 1777
Bournemouth BH5 1YR
Telephone 01270 772850
Support line 01235 772852

Benefits Enquiry Line
Freephone 0800 882200

Royal Society for the Prevention of Accidents
Cannon House
The Priory
Queensway
Birmingham
Telephone 0121 200 2000

Disability employment adviser:
Contact the local job centre.

Bibliography

Agurell, S., Berlin, A., Ferngren, H. *et al.* (1975). Plasma levels of diazepam after pareneteral and rectal administration in children. *Epilepsia,* **175,** 27–37.

Betts, T. (1998). *Epilepsy, Psychiatry and Learning Difficulty.* Martin Dunitz Ltd., UK. ISBN 1-85317-616-8.

British National Formulary (2001). British Medical Association.

Brown, S., Betts, T., Crawford, P. *et al.* (1998). Epilepsy needs revisited: revised epilepsy needs document for the UK. *Seizure,* **7,** 435–46. See also *Epilepsy, An Agenda for Action,* British Epilepsy Association, leaflet. http:www.bea-connect.com

Central Health Services Council (1969). Advisory committee on the health and welfare of handicapped people with epilepsy. Report of a Joint sub-committee of the standing medical advisory committee and the advisory committee on the health and welfare of handicapped persons (the Ried Report) London, HMSO.

Chadwick, D. and Usiskin, S. (1987). *Living with Epilepsy.* Macdonald Optima (reprinted 1994). ISBN 0-356-19676-3.

Chadwick, D., Orme, M., Appleton, R. *et al.* (1991). *The Management of Epilepsy in General Practice.* The Alden Press, Oxford. ISBN 0-948270-25X.

Chappell, B. and Crawford, P. (1999). *Epilepsy at your fingertips.* Class Publishing, London. ISBN 1-872362-51-6.

Clinical Standards Advisory Group (1999). *Services to People with Epilepsy.* Chair Professor Alison Kitson, Report prepared by Professor Simon Shorvon and others. Department of Health. ISBN 1-84182-12594.

Cockerell, O. and Shorvon, S. (1996). *Epilepsy: Current Concepts.* Current Medical Literature Ltd, London.

Department of Health (DoH) (1999). Review of prescribing,

supply and administration of medicines: final report. The Stationary Office, London.

Department of Health and Social Services (DHSS) (1983). Working group for people with epilepsy. HMSO, London.

Driving and Vehicle Licensing Agency (1999). *For Medical Practitioners, At a Glance Guide to the Current Medical Standards of Fitness to Drive*. Medical Division DVLA.

Duncan, J. S., Shorvon, S. D. and Fish, D. R. (1995). *Clinical Epilepsy*. Churchill Livingston, New York. ISBN 0443-04936-X.

Ellis, S. J. (1988). *Clinical Neurology: Essential Concepts*. Butterworth-Heinemann, Oxford. ISBN 0-7506-3343-3.

Elwes, R. D., Marshall, J., Beattie, A., Newman, P. K. (1991). Epilepsy and employment. A community-based survey in an area of high unemployment. *Journal of Neurology/neurosurgery and Psychiatry*, **54**(3), 200–203.

Epilepsy Task Force, UK Epilepsy Services Provision (1998). *A National Audit of Service*. EFT Secretariat, PO Box 16696, London, WC1A 2PD Tel: 020 7300 6300.

Epilepsy Task Force, Joint Epilepsy Council (1999). Service Development Kit. PO Box 16696, London, WC1A 2PD.

Fisher, R.S. and Handforth, A. (1999). Reassessment: Vagus nerve stimulation for epilepsy. Neurology, Vol. 53 (Special Article).

Guberman, A. and Bruni, J. (1999). *Essentials of Clinical Epilepsy*. Butterworth-Heinemann, USA. ISBN 0-7506-7109-2.

Hanscomb, A. and Hughes, L. (1999). *Epilepsy*. Ward Lock, London. ISBN 0-7063-7404-5.

Hollins, S., Bernal, J., Thacker, A. and Kopper, L. (1999). *Getting on with Epilepsy*. Books Without Words Series, Bell & Bain Ltd, UK. ISBN 1-901242-39-0.

Joint Epilepsy Council. *Epilepsy, Men and Sexual Dysfunction*, Leaflet (out of print).

Mills, N. L., Bachmann, M. O., Campbell, R. *et al.* (1999). Effects of a primary care based epilepsy specialist nurse service on quality of care from the patients' perspective: results at two-year follow-up. *Seizure*, **8(5),** 291–6.

Oxley, J. and Smith, J. (1991). *The Epilepsy Reference Book*. Faber and Faber Ltd, London. ISBN 0-571-16253-3.

Remy, C., Jourdil, N., Villemain, D. *et al.* (1992). Intrarectal diazepam in epileptic adults. *Epilepsia*, **33**(2), 353–8.

Ried, S. and Beck-Mannagetta, G. (1996). *Epilepsy, Pregnancy and the Child*. Blackwell Wissenschaft, Berlin. ISBN 0-632-04164-1.

Russell, A. (1998). *Health Care Assistants Guide to Epilepsy*. Unison Education & Training. Available from the National Society for Epilepsy.

Sander, J. W. and Hart, Y. M. (1999). *Epilepsy: Questions and Answers*. Merti Publishing International, UK. ISBN 1-873413-80-7.

Scally, G. and Donaldson, L. J. (1998) Clinical governance and drive for quality improvement in the New NHS in England. *BMJ*, **317**, 61–5.

Service Development Kit, Epilepsy Task Force, Joint Epilepsy Council, PO Box 16696, London, WC1A 2PD.

Shorvon, S. (2000). *Handbook of Epilepsy Treatment*. Blackwell Science Ltd. ISBN 0-632-04849-2.

Stephen, J. L. and Brodie, M. (2000). Epilepsy in elderly people. *Lancet*, **355**, 1441–6.

Taylor, M. P. (1996). *Managing Epilepsy in Primary Care*. Blackwell Science, Oxford. ISBN 0-86542-972-3.

The Disability Discrimination Act (1996). *Access to Goods, Facilities and Services*. HMSO, DL80, April. ISBN 0-11-270955-9.

UKCC (1993). *Standards for Records and Record Keeping*, http://www.ukcc.org.uk

UKCC (1992a). *Code of Professional Conduct*, http://www.ukcc.org.uk

UKCC (1992b). *The Scope of Professional Practice*, http://www.ukcc.org.uk

World Health Organization (1997). Fact Sheet No. 165. WHO Press Office, http://www.who

Index